The Cancer Experience

The Cancer Experience

The Doctor, the Patient, the Journey

Roy B. Sessions

ROWMAN & LITTLEFIELD PUBLISHERS, INC.
Lanham • Boulder • New York • Toronto • Plymouth, UK

Published by Rowman & Littlefield Publishers, Inc.
A wholly owned subsidiary of The Rowman & Littlefield Publishing Group, Inc.
4501 Forbes Boulevard, Suite 200, Lanham, Maryland 20706
http://www.rowmanlittlefield.com

Estover Road, Plymouth PL6 7PY, United Kingdom

British Library Cataloguing in Publication Information Available

Library of Congress Cataloging-in-Publication Data

Sessions, Roy B.
    The cancer experience : the doctor, the patient, the journey / Roy B. Sessions.
      p. cm.
    ISBN 978-1-4422-1621-1 (cloth : alk. paper)— ISBN 978-1-4422-1623-5 (ebook)
    1. Cancer—Psychological aspects. 2. Cancer—Patients—Care—Moral and ethical
aspects. I. Title.
    RC263.S445 2012
    616.99′4—dc23   2011047812

♾™ The paper used in this publication meets the minimum requirements of
American National Standard for Information Sciences—Permanence of Paper
for Printed Library Materials, ANSI/NISO Z39.48-1992.

Printed in the United States of America

Dedicated to those brave patients
who have taken *The Journey*.

Contents

Author's Note on Terminology

I have taken the liberty of using certain words interchangeably, not to invite inconsistency, but to add variability to the text. The words *physician* and *doctor* are used almost interchangeably, with the exception being that those of our colleagues who have graduated from schools of osteopathy, have the designated degree of doctors of osteopathy (DO) and are referred to as doctor but not physician. Those who have graduated from medical schools receive an MD, and are called either doctor or physician. In this text, therefore, a referring doctor can be either a doctor of osteopathy or a medical doctor, that is, a physician.

The words *oncologist, cancer physician,* and *cancer doctor* all denote medical doctors with a particular focus or special training in the management of tumors, benign as well as malignant. The word *oncologist* is generic, and can refer to a surgical oncologist, a radiation oncologist, a medical oncologist, or a psycho-oncologist. Surgical oncologists are further subdivided, but because this book concerns cancer in general those distinctions are not relevant here. Suffice it to say that in all of the surgical oncology specialties there is the commonality of interest in and focus on cancer, usually to the exclusion of other diseases of the various body systems. Thus, the word *oncology* is used throughout the book in a generic way. Medical oncologists are sometimes referred to as chemotherapists.

Finally, the words *cancer* and *malignancy* are the same, while *tumor* is a general word that includes both benign and malignant growths.

Foreword

$\mathcal{N}$o medical diagnosis is more fearsome than the diagnosis of cancer. The very mention of the word is enough to trigger a confluence of physical, emotional, spiritual, and financial crises. The resulting maelstrom of life-changing events engulfs patients, their families, and their doctors. If the cancer involves the head and neck, fear of physical disfigurement augments the patient's dread of alienation from the world of purposeful existence.

In this book, Dr. Roy Sessions reflects on his life as a dedicated head and neck surgeon living daily within the disrupting milieu of his patients' cancer. He describes how cancer confronted and challenged his own technical and personal resources as a professed healer. Sometimes he cured, sometimes ameliorated or palliated. All too often, he traveled with his patient along the path of human finitude to the patient's death.

Repeatedly, Sessions recognizes the need to join surgical and medical competence with the capacity to enter into the patient's real-world predicament, and for this a strong bond of trust is essential. He laments the weakening of trust between physicians and patients in the contemporary world. Without trust it is difficult for a physician to be healer, helper, and friend. Without trust it is difficult to sustain patient and doctor in their journey through the cancer experience.

Sessions lays a good part of the responsibility to build the requisite trust on the physician. To be authentic this trust must proceed from the physician's personal dedication to the primacy of the patient's welfare. To be authentic this trust must rest on a moral commitment. Dr. Sessions outlines his own moral commitment in terms of the traditional Hippocratic ethic. Thus he expresses unapologetic opposition to inducing the death of patients. For him the legalization of assisted suicide is the "dark side" of end-of-life care in patients with cancer. There is a fine line between a physician helping a patient die and actually inducing death. He fears that the growing economic strictures on the care of dying patients will hasten the push to death in cancer victims.

This is a book replete with clinical wisdom earned through the author's dedication to the care of some of medicine's most desperately ill patients. It will be of interest and instructional value to medical students, aspiring and practicing oncologists—medical, surgical, radiation—as well as physicians generally. But Sessions intends his book for the general public as well. Importantly, he makes the case that a better understanding of doctors by patients and their families is beneficial for all concerned. The cases Sessions describe will resonate with our own experiences or those of our families and friends. His thoughts extend well beyond the cancer experience to include other serious life-threatening trauma and illness.

Some may disagree with the author's firm adhesion to the traditional norms of professional ethics. Few however can deny the moral nature of medical practice for anyone who "professes" to be a healer. Medical students, those "physicians in utero," should ponder the author's unrelenting moral commitment to the patient's welfare. As we approach the revolutionary changes now occurring in the way we care for patients, we need to be reminded that all our efforts must finally be channeled toward the help and relief of a human in distress. Anyone who "professes" to possess the requisite knowledge to heal must use it to the advantage of the one who seeks and needs it.

The "final common pathway" of the doctor's effort is the good of the patient. This is its moral lever. Current proposals for evidence-based, personalized, value-based, or systems care must traverse this ancient pathway if it is to be morally justified. The sick will always need physicians who practice technically correct, humanely administered, and morally guided personal care. Sessions's book provides the compass that must not be lost in the current zeal for change in how physicians and society care for the sick, the most vulnerable of our fellow citizens.

Edmund D. Pellegrino, MD, MACP
Professor Emeritus of Medicine and Medical Ethics, Georgetown University
and Interim Director, Center for Clinical Bioethics,
Georgetown University Medical Center

Acknowledgments

$\mathcal{I}$n developing this book, I attempted to address both the medical and lay public by finding a lexicon that both camps would be comfortable with. In seeking this balance, it was difficult to avoid the inadvertent tilt toward what was comfortable and familiar—in my case toward the world of the cancer caregivers. Realizing this natural tendency prompted me to "field test" the preliminary manuscript on nonmedical people, several of whom had been cancer patients, and who happened to be educated and critical individuals.

Since psychosocial matters run throughout the corpus of my writing, it seemed presumptuous to promote my ideas without the scrutiny of experts in the psychiatry world. Likewise, the legal implications and facts within my story made it imperative that scholars in that arena read the manuscript. I also asked several practicing physicians to critically read and critically suggest. Finally, the bioethical implications of the book's theme were addressed by one of the preeminent scholars in that world. Essentially all of these individuals had free reign to either encourage or squelch further development.

I am deeply appreciative for the intense analysis of two colleagues, both of whom are professors of psychiatry at the Georgetown University School of Medicine: Stephen Green and Richard Goldberg are both very busy men who showed real generosity by somehow finding the time to study the manuscript. They are both noted authors in their own academic spheres. Their guidance and encouragement provided the spark for me to continue the project.

Two extraordinarily articulate and intelligent individuals, Christopher O'Flin, and the late Ambassador Stephan Minikes poked, tweaked, and critiqued my writing with the precision and methodical manner of legal scholars. Their enthusiasm for the content encouraged me to believe that there really was a nonmedical readership for the book.

Asking colleagues to commit valuable time from a busy internal medicine practice to read an esoteric manuscript is no small request: so it was with my colleague, Doctor Michael Newman, who did exactly that while on his vacation, after which he came back with tough questions and suggestions—most of which were in some way incorporated in the next draft. I thank Doctor Charles Cummings of Johns Hopkins School of Medicine for his appraisal and advice. My former boss at Baylor College of Medicine and a mentor, Doctor Bob Alford, an icon in the academic world, graciously read and appraised my text and made suggestions that helped immensely.

Finally, Professor Edmund Pellegrino, the noted Georgetown scholar and former chairman of the President's Commission on Bioethics was the first to encourage the development of the rudimentary thoughts that were restlessly swirling about in my mind. I thank him for his early critique of my work, and for providing the foreword to the completed text.

The tedium of manuscript and bibliographic preparation cannot be overestimated. I am grateful to Anita Cheslek for the patience and attention to details that are essential to a refined final product. My copyeditor, Gary J. Hamel, made sense, gave rhythm, and generally helped to create efficient writing out of occasional literary chaos. I thank him for his precision and thoroughness—both the product and the author have been enhanced as a result.

Lastly, I thank my most demanding critic and strongest advocate, my wife, Mary Cousart Sessions, who convinced me that retirement was really only about shifting gears by starting new intellectual pursuits and retaining my enthusiasm for being a teacher. Fundamental, but so true!

Roy B. Sessions
Charleston, SC

I

INTELLECTUAL CONSIDERATIONS

Prologue

$\mathcal{T}$his book promotes my philosophy about a number of what I consider to be important matters—some derived from common sense, others more transcendental—that relate to the central theme of cancer. It is predictable that the credibility of what I have written will be scrutinized by those that nod in the affirmative as well as others that scoff at my audacity in attempting to tackle these sometimes weighty subjects—I hope that the former outnumber the latter. It's for others to judge whether thirty-plus years of surgical oncology qualifies me to undertake this—obviously I believe that it does. Even though my intention was to avoid writing a memoir, I suppose my avoidance was not absolute, since I have borrowed extensively on my personal professional experiences in order to make certain points.

What you will read is a series of thoughts and reflections based on memories from a professional lifetime of taking care of cancer patients. In seeking to avoid the memoir label, I suppose I was defensively protecting against reveling in self, impaired by the delusion that my personal story would be as interesting to others as it is to me. So perhaps it is a memoir of sorts, or perhaps not—after all, it's only a label. With that ambiguity conceded, I would ask the reader to believe that this work is not about me, but rather about occurrences and matters that have helped to define me. Granted, there is a degree of audacity inherent in the persona of most surgeons: more than just being willing to invade the body, surgeons actually seek out and even savor that intense responsibility. As a surgeon, I am guilty of that mind-set, but it is my hope that neither vanity nor audacity is the catalyst for this book. So I ask the indulgence of the reader during the few early paragraphs that relate to my background.

There are three reasons why a brief recounting of my background seemed important to the mission of the book. First of all, nonfiction, whether addressed to a medical or a nonmedical audience, often reflects the author's perspective, and when I read such work, I like to have some knowledge of the person promoting their thoughts. I realize that the material is there for me to accept or not, but I am more comfortable in deciding its value if I can visualize the author. Secondly, it is my hope that the young doctors who read this book will be influenced by my unabashed career passion, and that they will be inspired to let their emotions fly freely in seeking to realize fantasies and dreams. The third purpose for the references to my background is that it is important for medical and lay readers alike to understand the profession's evolution, especially as it pertains to certain critical themes of this writing, such as the role of physicians in our society—past and present—and the appreciation by both groups of the enormity of the responsibilities doctors assume in dealing with cancer patients, most of whom have extraordinary needs.

Influences on My Development

Without the passion, it's only a profession.

—*Lucian Radu Sulica, MD (1967–)*

As I have grown older, perhaps even "grown up," I have come to realize my good fortune in knowing at a young age what I wanted my life's work to be. As early as junior high school, I somehow realized that I wanted to be a physician. When this first dawned on me is unclear. Almost certainly it wasn't a sudden revelation. Truth be known, I don't really remember ever wanting to do anything else. Whenever its beginning, what was to become an obsession to achieve that lofty goal grew in a continuous crescendo—first modestly, then progressively more dominant—finally taking charge of me. By the time of high school graduation, I had reached the next level in which fantasies about being a surgeon—not just a doctor—occupied my thoughts. I am now embarrassed to think how throughout college, I must have bored many friends with plans that no matter how exciting to me, undoubtedly tested their tolerance. Later during medical school, as I was introduced to the different specialties, my primary field of interest changed many times, but as I progressed through the clinical curriculum, even though I loved it all, the pathway always returned to surgery. During medical school, I was continuously—"twenty-four, seven"—surrounded by people who were equally consumed, and the talk that probably had bored my college friends was usually the topic de jour. The commonality shared by most of us was a totality of desire to transform our fantasies into reality.

As with many obsessions, the source of the underlying passion is often inexplicable. While I can't speak for others equally obsessed, I can at least speculate on what helped to invigorate me. Certain family traditions and members had probably influenced me to some degree. For instance, my

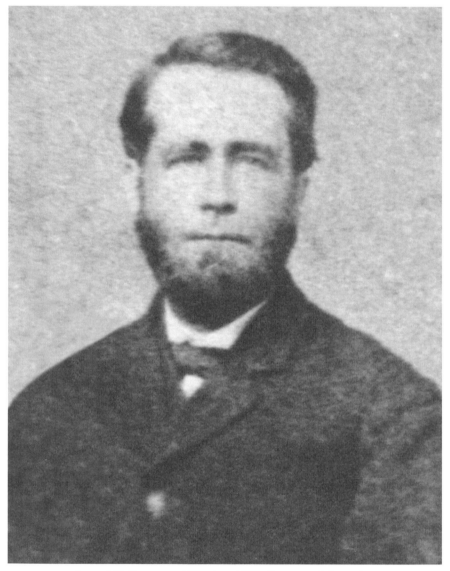

Samuel G. Compton, MD, circa 1875. Courtesy of the author.

great-grandfather, Samuel Gilbert Compton, MD, had been a surgeon in the Army of Virginia during the Civil War, and the story of his exploits was the stuff of family legend. Perhaps he was a part of the motivation, despite the fact that he died long before I came on the scene. However, my reference to Doctor Compton by name is not so much as it pertains to my inner motivational force, but instead it is to use him as a basis of comparison for the discussion of certain issues covered in the early part of the book. So reader, please make note of my ancestor's name, because it will resurface later in this writing.

A more significant influence on my career passion probably was my contact with a great uncle, Oliver Perry Daly, MD, who had been a noted surgeon in New Orleans. Although my interaction with him occurred when I was a schoolboy and he had already retired, the atmosphere around this man was electric for me. One would have thought that he had discovered fire or invented the wheel. I would wager that had he been aware of my adulation and awe he would have been embarrassed. Like most surgeons, Doctor Daly was not the model of humility, but he was a good man who exemplified the correct reasons for being a physician—and certainly realistic enough not to have claimed to be the iconic figure that I felt him to be. Later, during my many years in the academic surgical world, whenever I interacted with young aspirants to the profession—medical students, interns, and residents—my memory of Doctor Daly served to remind me of my responsibilities as a role model. Although he died sometime ago, my memories of him are vivid, and I think he would have been pleased by his positive effect on me.

In admitting my idol worship of this man, it occurs to me that educational paternalism is actually an important part of my motivation for writing this book—not the sort of paternalism founded in condescension, but rather that which evolves from traditional values and a sense of obligation to the profession. Much the same as being a parent, the academic physician's[1] responsibility in this regard cannot be overstated; the ethics and morality that we bring to the table—the example we set—has a real impact on the next generation of doctors. Make no mistake about it, they watch and they listen. It is my hope that this book will help to ingrain a mind-set in young doctors that it's the norm rather than the exception for a physician—especially one devoted to cancer patients—to think and act according to moral and ethical standards. In point of fact, I have always thought that moral and ethical behavior is an integral part of the larger package of human qualities that all physicians ought to possess.

I have diverged somewhat from my description of the influences on my development. Even though Doctor Daly's impact on me was undoubtedly real, my obsession with becoming a physician was not that simple. The desire to be a doctor is vocational—it resides in one's bone marrow—relentless and domineering—and when one is asked to explain it, words tend to fail. A vocation, unlike an avocation, is neither temporary nor ever whimsical—essentially, a true vocation is a force of nature that when not compartmentalized can lead to personal calamity. There was a time when, like a young bride-to-be preoccupied with an impending marriage, I daydreamed constantly about being a member of the medical guild. My attitude when I went through the medical school selection process—in which thousands apply but only one to two hundred are admitted to the typical freshman class—was that "if they just let me in, I'll study twenty-three hours a day in order to stay in." Fortunately, I was admitted, and thankfully, I didn't have to study twenty-three hours a day, even though it seemed so at the time. With continuous family support and encouragement, I was able to focus on the intense curriculum, and after a rocky start and a huge adjustment, I went on to graduate. As it turned out, this milestone was only the beginning of an extraordinary lifelong journey of education, emotional responsibilities, and rigorous demands, most of which yielded a bountiful harvest of gratification and rewards and only few regrets.

Medical school graduation was followed by a one-year internship, then a two-year tour as a United States Naval Medical Officer, and finally, a long residency. Then, "all of a sudden," I was on my own as a surgeon. Actually, it's a stretch to claim professional solitude at that time, because with my first academic appointment, I became part of the faculty of a medical school and was on the staff of a major medical center. There I was among wise and experienced fellow surgeons whose maturity and judgment were of immeasurable value to me.

Even though my focus on cancer didn't start until ten years after training was completed, it was to become the work that consumed me for over thirty years. Why I gravitated to that world is not easy to explain; perhaps it was because I thought cancer surgery to be technically the most challenging, and perhaps I also thought the impact of this work on people's lives was the most profound. Most agree that the physical and emotional needs of cancer patients are extraordinary, and whether true or not, I felt that being a cancer physician was somehow more important than anything else in medicine. For reasons that probably include that demanding companion called vanity, I wanted to do something really important—something that enhanced humankind. Thomas Jefferson envisioned the development of a "natural" (Jefferson's word) American aristocracy that was based on pluck, achievement, excellence, and the drive to improve the human condition, rather than on social status, inheritance, or wealth.[2] His goals were music to my ears, and I wanted to be part of such an aristocracy. I thought then, and think now, that there is no better pathway to achieve these goals than in the medical profession.

· 2 ·

Why the Book?

The entirety of this particular *why* is elusive. Probably, the answer lies in a medley of emotions, many of which result from a deep affection for and a sense of responsibility to this most extraordinary profession; and I suspect the emotions have been within me for sometime. The title could have been simply "Reflections on Medicine and Oncology," but that seemed too passive to evoke the vital importance of what we do, and steady confidence in that seems more important now than ever. For years, I have practiced medicine with the enemy being a disease; now however, the enemy list must include nebulous change that is being enacted by thoughtless and shortsighted people who seek to make doctors less than special. I view this book as a vehicle with which to expound—without rambling, I hope—on a variety of issues important to mitigating change so that those values that make medicine a singular profession are retained. That quest, therefore, ought to be part of the *why*.

Fundamental to the philosophy that I have developed as I have matured is the realization that being a physician is a privilege and that it does in fact involve a higher calling—a vocation, if you will—and with it a sober responsibility to the community of humankind. Caring for cancer patients further intensifies that responsibility because the typical patient, frightened and vulnerable, justifiably expects a commitment to excellence, a seriousness of purpose, compassion for those served, and an ethos of integrity and humanity from the cancer team in general and the cancer physician in particular. With cancer, the demands imposed on the physician are greater, and whether justifiably or not, the stakes are perceived to be higher than with other illnesses. Those in the profession who accept these responsibilities are to be saluted, because this is, and should involve, a serious lifestyle, with little room for frivolity or casualness. At a minimum, dilettantish physicians who value style over substance should not be welcomed into the oncology specialties. Obviously, style and substance are not mutually exclusive, but in the world of cancer care, the former must be substantially subordinated to the latter. Promotion of professional sobriety is yet another component of the *why*.

Within this book, therefore, there is much for doctors (especially cancer doctors) as well as the lay public, cancer victims and their families in particular. It is my hope that readers who are medical students, residents, and other young physicians possess an intrinsic desire to hang on to the youthful idealism and chastity of thought with which they entered the educational cascade that leads to a degree in medicine, and postdoctoral training in oncology. The tenacity of purpose required at these early stages is derived largely from appropriate motivation, and because of this, the innocent exuberance of youth should be nurtured and respected by the "elders." Mentors who harbor cynicism, whether justified or not, should refrain from spewing negativity; better they suffer silently than encourage the insidious depletion of youthful vim. The number of physicians' children who apply to medical school has diminished in recent times, and this fact suggests that cynicism has already taken a toll to some degree. For those lay readers, whether they be cancer victims or not, my hope is that this book will allow them to develop a better understanding of those physicians who devote their lives to the care of this dreaded disease, and by better understanding them, to appreciate the value of a partnership between physicians and the public in a common cause.

That this book is focused on the subject of cancer is not a coincidence, for it is within this world that I have spent most of my professional life. In truth, however, much of what I write relates to medicine in general, and the underlying cancer theme is in some respects a base for making certain generic points. With that concession granted, however, I believe it's safe to say that the ideals and responsibilities of which I write are particularly relevant to the world of cancer medicine, both from the physician's perspective as well as the patient's. To some degree, this writing attempts to describe the life of cancer physicians by means of exploring the psyche of cancer patients.[1] In doing that, I have emphasized the all important physician-patient link that makes caring for these patients a unique experience in medicine. Perhaps patients and their families who read this book will also benefit by better understanding the other side of the physician-patient equation. By realizing the intensity and the emotional nature of the life of an oncologist, a patient or family member might be able to more easily reconcile various frustrations encountered during the tortuous and scary journey through diagnosis and treatment of this disease. Finally, by my using this approach, aspirants to the oncology specialties might better realize that to perform in this arena is neither an ordinary responsibility nor an ordinary commitment; none in medicine should be, but with cancer, there truly is heightened passion and drama.

I undertake this writing in the autumn of my life, which is a time when one has the luxury of being able to reflect and evaluate, a time for pondering professional and personal successes and failures, a time for realizing how many issues that seemed so important during one's youth are not what real gratification is about. Essentially it is a time for understanding that a person's most treasured legacies ought to be about kindness, service, education, generosity, and having set and maintained lofty standards for one's children and protégées to emulate. Although wisdom doesn't automatically come with gray hair, with some exceptions, the full appreciation of life's revelations are more within the dominion of the mature. Could it be that these ideals and principles are what the previously mentioned Jeffersonian natural aristocracy is really all about? I do believe that to be so—even though I seem to have inadvertently wandered into that zone of idealism without actually calling it or even recognizing it by name. In the prologue of his 1967 autobiography— that too written in the autumn of life—Bertrand Russell claimed that three passions, simple but overwhelmingly strong, had governed his life: the longing for love, the search for knowledge, and pity for the suffering of mankind.[2] While I would question the limitation of his list, the point is well taken and pertains to the mission statement of the medical profession

To state what will become obvious, I have taken considerable literary liberty throughout this book. After a lifetime of a very busy medical practice, I have developed strong opinions and attitudes about patient care, some of which are undoubtedly not shared by some colleagues. However, I believe my ways of doing and thinking are correct—for me, at least, they have been effective. Certainly, at this stage of my life I don't hesitate to put my thoughts out there for public scrutiny, hoping to help cancer patients understand physicians better and, on the other hand, to aid physicians in dealing with patients. In response to those who take umbrage with my doing this, I believe I am indulging in one of the privileges afforded to those who are aging—one is expected to become opinionated, and perhaps even dogmatic. To borrow from the logic and the humor of Sir Winston Churchill, if such is not my right, it ought to be![3] Humor aside, what I write is based on what has worked for me in finding a balanced approach in guiding and treating thousands of cancer patients over thirty years. Because much of the content of this book is based in part on common sense, my own values, and my life's experiences, it is, unlike my prior contributions to the medical literature, not really a medical book; instead it represents a consideration of various themes that subjectively swirl around the periphery of medical care—delving into human interaction, motivation, idealism, mental and physical suffering, and even touching on the transcendental zones of mortality and spiritualism.

Specific cancer therapy plans are intentionally excluded from this writing; instead, my intent is to stimulate a thoughtful discussion of emotional and practical matters that beset cancer patients and their physicians. I have drawn on science indirectly, but more of what I have written has come from extensive experiences in the clinical arena, and as a result, I have utilized a number of patient-based anecdotes, all of which were recalled with as much accuracy as the passage of time allowed. The patient stories are, by and large, real, but on several occasions I have used hypothetical situations, and I have stated that where it is the case. I have known a number of cancer physicians who, despite having developed a vast reservoir of practical pearls and experiences, went to their graves not having documented much of their real clinical wisdom; hence, what they have taught verbally is what survives them. In saying this, I acknowledge the extraordinary value of what is known in medical parlance as "bedside teaching." Simply put, my goal in this endeavor is to immortalize some of my practical wisdom—not necessarily knowledge, which is somewhat different.

Keeping these matters in mind, I will pose key questions: What should a cancer patient reasonably expect of the system, the cancer team, and especially, the cancer physician? What should a cancer physician be able to expect of the patient? What are the physician's responsibilities to the patient—to the family? How much information about the disease is enough; how much is too much; and importantly, how much is too little? Where do optimism and encouragement end and the gravitas of pragmatism and realism begin? How specific and how graphic should the doctor be? Is pessimism allowed, and if so, should it be shared with the patient? How forcefully should the case be made for the recommended treatment; that is to say, should the physician attempt to alter the patient's search for autonomy when they are disinclined to follow the physician's recommendations? What is the cancer physician's role when treatment fails, or when no treatment is given because of the advanced state of the disease? How important are quality of life and quality of death; and specifically, what is the cancer physician's role in the dying process? Is death solely within the dominion of spiritual forces, or is there a place for the physician as a taker of life—that is to say, the catalyst to death? And if not an active player, should a physician even introduce the possibility of patient-induced death, that is, suicide? The oath that we have lived by clearly says "No" to the taking of life by the physician, but should this part of the oath be adapted "in search of modern relevance"? That certainly has happened in several European countries, and in three states in America (Washington, Oregon, and Montana), in which there are laws condoning varying degrees of physician involvement with induced patient death. Finally, because of the natural instinct for self-protection, is it justified for the cancer physician to remain emotionally detached, and in doing that, not provide an intensity of feeling that might be more helpful to the patient during treatment and even on into the dying process?

These questions and many others randomly flow through the lexicology of cancer management. The answers often cannot be rigid because so much of human nature varies from individual to individual—patient and physician alike—and there should be a somewhat tailored approach for the individual patient. With that said, however, a pattern of consistency ideally should underlie it all, and the standards by which all of these questions are answered should be set by a medical profession that understands and advocates what is right as opposed to what is wrong.

· 3 ·

Protecting What's Good through the Educational Process: Capitalizing on the Gene Pool

He plants trees to benefit another generation.

—Caecilius Statius, quoted by Cicero

The integrity of any profession is largely dependent on selecting the right applicants—in our case physicians generally and oncologists specifically— and then building on character and values. During the ten years when I was chairman of a surgical department at Georgetown University Medical School, in Washington, D.C., I directed a residency training program, the corps of which consisted of eighteen young doctors (three per year, in a six-year curriculum), all of whom had been carefully selected during a very competitive process from a large pool of highly qualified medical students. Most of the applicants were extraordinary, having excelled in academics, in sports, community service, and so on. Had we relied on these accomplishments alone, the selection could have been accomplished by drawing lots. Essentially, they were all smart and multidimensional people; so the three were chosen each year largely by relying on qualities of character and a value system that included morality, ethical behavior, family values, patriotism, integrity, willingness to subordinate the interest of the individual to that of the group, absolute academic honesty as well as a willingness to adhere to an honor code, a commitment to excellence, a desire to be of service to humankind, and a love of the profession. I don't claim that we were always correct in our judgment of the candidates, but our batting average was quite good.

I fervently believe that the perpetuation of high ethical and moral standards by means of careful recruitment is the single most important responsibility of the profession's leadership; and the opportunity for success in this endeavor is present because the talent pool from which to choose is populated by young men and women already imbued with these qualities and

14

values. Educators should commit to the notion that with the correct selection process for advanced training, and then by the imposition of the highest expectations and standards on those selected, the ideals recurring in the themes of this book are achievable in the next generation of cancer doctors. In molding young physicians, and particularly future oncologists, it's essential to select those who respond in a positive way to the emphasis on character and values. This is no simple task, because in attempting to be modern—dare I admit it, politically correct—whether by exclusion or otherwise, we have de-emphasized these basic principles in our guidance of young people through the minefields of today's world; and I believe that, in the process, they have suffered from an insidious intellectual and moral debilitation that results from lowered expectations. I have never been reluctant to discuss important professional and even personal values in meetings with my residents; and it has always gratified me how well this generation responds to these "old-fashioned ideas." The truth is, while these values can be applied to many endeavors in life, they are especially relevant to the medical profession, and in fact, should form its very foundation. To carry this notion even further, I believe it's especially important in the world of cancer medicine, where so much value comes from interpersonal chemistry between the physician and patient.

I owe much to the residents that I have selected and helped to train. Their expectations of me have provided a behavioral compass throughout my professional life, and our interaction is embedded in the infrastructure of my clinical philosophy. Importantly, this generation of young physicians has given me a sense of optimism for the future of medicine as well as a reason to sustain enthusiasm for teaching.

Considering the array of issues that influence the practice of medicine—political turmoil, socioeconomic uncertainty, changing value systems of people in general, and so on—it's not surprising that in this country there is an atmosphere of concern for the dynamic target that we euphemistically refer to as the Health Care System. In fact, it's an understatement to say that major uncertainty and insecurity exist in all of society about the future of American medicine. While I also have concerns for the system, I do have steady confidence in the intelligence, the goodness, and the quality of the next generations of physicians. They truly are the cream of the crop in our culture, and an important goal of the leadership of the government, the profession, and the insurance industry should be to create a consumer-friendly and functional health care system that does not squelch the optimism and idealism of the future keepers of the public's health. A preliminary analysis of this statement is particularly relevant to this book, as I will discuss at some length the emotional burden of taking care of cancer patients—and when that burden is added to the cumbersome daily chores that physicians face today, we should all be concerned. To paraphrase Thomas Smith, the professor and chair of Hematology, Oncology, and Palliative Care at Virginia Commonwealth University, oncology is already very hard work, and with increasing resistance to higher reimbursements for cancer care, it is no wonder that the United States faces a looming 40 percent shortage of oncologists.[1] There are a variety of reasons why so many outstanding young people have historically been willing to undergo the long, grueling, and very expensive period of training required to become a physician. That the academic elite of our young people will continue to have this affinity for the profession cannot be taken for granted, however. We should not ignore the benefits that have hitherto served to offset their very demanding education and lifestyle. When the negatives start to outweigh the positives, many will seek other avenues for their idealism and ingenuity.

· 4 ·

Oncology Is Not for the Emotionally Stingy

For unto whomsoever much is given, of him shall be much required; and to whom men have committed much, of him they will ask the more.

—Luke 12:48

*B*ecause repeatedly witnessing agony and death can be emotionally erosive, the personal price paid by the cancer doctor is substantial. On the other hand, many of the 2010 treatment strategies with which we attack this enemy are successful, and the rewards seem to consistently replenish the corpus of our spirit. The ebb and flow of one's feelings is not always predictable, however, because there are certain patients for whom a cancer doctor develops real love—totally within the bounds of propriety, of course—which runs deeper than the average professional concern. An interesting book, *Doctoring*, by Eric Cassell articulates this vulnerability that is shared by many physicians.[1] This circumstance can lead to an involuntary reciprocal response that I believe is a subconscious means of self-protection from sadness and emotional pain. It is intuitively understandable, therefore, why doctors—especially cancer doctors—often unintentionally shield themselves emotionally by being remote from their patients. Isn't that so with many human relationships in which love and affection are withheld because of fear? I now realize that I was emotionally stingy with patients in the youthful stages of my career. With maturation, however, I came to realize that the real emotional "juice" for a physician comes from the bonding and the affection that one has earlier sought to avoid. At the risk of seeming melodramatic, as I grew emotionally, I came to realize that it is a gift to have the opportunity to interface with cancer patients and to reap the rewards of success—not by always conquering the disease, mind you, because unfortunately such is not the case—but by finding

17

the human connection that helps guide and support patients in their time of extreme need. It has always amazed me how much genuine affection and gratitude cancer patients are capable of doling out. So when friends remark that it must be discouraging to be a cancer physician, I make the point that while emotionally taxing and often depressing, quite the opposite of discouraging is the norm. I almost feel guilty for experiencing such gratification that is indirectly a product of another person's misfortune. A physician does not reach this plane of nirvana, however, without bravely discarding the shield that prevents the penetration of those emotional juices. Absent this commitment, both the patient and the physician suffer. In point of fact, for the latter, failure to commit can lead to crippling professional unhappiness. It is my unscientific observation that some of the most morose and unhappy physicians are those who care for cancer patients without having the emotional connection that I am talking about.

Those seemingly unemotional colleagues who behave in this fashion out of self-protectiveness hopefully will eventually mature out of that state, as I did. But I have known cancer specialists who, because they are emotionally barren, offer little empathy or affection, subliminally or otherwise. Some physicians simply lack the capacity for empathy toward others; therefore, they don't connect with the patient within that realm. They are unable to grieve or even inwardly shed tears in the patient's darkest hours. Such physicians go through the motions of compassion and interaction with patients largely through monologue and rote recitation of explanations and plans—often only for legal reasons. All the while they are surrounded by the emotional protection of frequent interruptions, a frantic schedule, and piles of technical and statistical details that leave the patient only mathematical probabilities and other analytical gauges with which to find hope.

Recently, I read a book entitled *Because Cowards Get Cancer Too*, in which the noted author, John Diamond, describes his own travails that resulted from successful cancer treatment. In the introduction, the author begrudgingly offers an oblique compliment to the profession by alluding to the medical orthodoxy that had performed well on his behalf, "despite all of its arrogance and self-serving smugness."[2] I was annoyed at first, and in a slight rush of defensiveness, thought him ungrateful; however, an incident from my past popped into my mind in which I had viewed physician behavior that mimicked exactly that same arrogance and smugness.

I remember as if it were yesterday that I had been embarrassed on behalf of the profession and felt advocacy for the patient. When telling tales from one's past, there is sometimes a tendency to overdramatize things, but in this instance, the memory is unembellished, and is as embarrassing today as it was thirty years ago. I had overheard a highly regarded colleague—a cancer surgeon of substantial reputation—respond to a frightened patient's desperate query of, "Doctor, do you think I have a chance to live through this?" by shrugging and impatiently saying in a cavalier manner, "How can I answer that? I'm not God, you know." As I witnessed this scene, I was struck by the insensitivity of his dismissive response to this penetrating question! It would have been so easy for him to hold the patient's arm while saying something like, "Mr. Wilson (to pick a name), that's a tough one to answer, but you know what, we'll give it our best shot, and with a little luck, and maybe a little help from higher sources, I think you have a real chance." Such a statement would have allowed the doctor to avoid a specific quantitative prediction while also giving the patient some hope.

Unfortunately, I have witnessed other similar physician-patient interchanges over the years, and I have come to believe that a cancer physician's unwillingness to invest him- or herself emotionally often stymies the development of true hope in patients. In my opinion, the capacity and the willingness to take such an emotional step are key ingredients of the profile of the effective oncologist; and students who are considering this avenue of study should think long and hard about both their ability and their willingness to invest the psychic energy necessary to function effectively in this field of endeavor. Importantly, can they accept the inevitable vulnerability that accompanies such an investment? Even after successful treatment, these patients have subliminal fears and lingering anxieties that can haunt them. A former colleague of mine, Doctor Sidney Winawer, professor of medicine at Memorial Sloan-Kettering Cancer Center in New York City, has aptly referred to this as "the black box of emotional turmoil that reverberates in the minds of cancer patients and their families."[3] Their need for the repeated reassurance of cancer's absence can be insatiable.

I have countless memories of cancer patients' dependency and need for reassurance, but I am reminded of one patient in particular. I treated a patient I will call J.R. in 1984, when I was a surgeon at one of New York City's great institutions, Memorial Sloan-Kettering Cancer Center. Mr. R. was a homegrown and quintessential New Yorker who had worked his way up through the ranks of the small business scene. He also happened to be a great guy. He had become a successful businessman through a combination of toughness, moxie, and hard work. Lacking formal education, his considerable wisdom was gained on the job and in life. J.R. had been referred to me with a moderately advanced cancer of the larynx. Fortunately, I was able to do a voice-sparing operation, and within a month or so after the conclusion of his treatment, he returned to a very active business life. My routine follow-up with such a patient had for many years been a ritual that consisted of reexamination each month of the first year after treatment, every two months during and until the end of the second year, every three months during and until the end of the third year, and then every six months from thereon. The reason for the long-term follow-up was practical—despite cure, people who have one head-and-neck cancer have a higher likelihood of developing a second cancer in the same general area at some point in the future. This continued observation is designed for early detection of such a cancer. As a bonus, such a follow-up also provides long-term reassurance for the patient. Some patients need more emotional attention than others, and in that regard, J.R. represented the extreme. I was able to switch him to the two-month exam periods, but he insisted on coming back every two months for years. Moving to a three-month schedule was a major event for him, and we stuck with that for almost ten more years. Eventually we got into a twice-a-year routine, but it took substantial persuasion on my part. No matter how much I reassured him, he was always worried about the return of the original cancer. Even after fifteen years of favorable checkups, he came in with a head of emotional steam, having spent the three or four days prior to the office visit building a gradual crescendo of anxiety and sleeplessness. On a number of occasions, he openly wept upon hearing the good news of a clear check.

I tell this story not to question this man's courage—which was uncontestable in most matters; he was a tough guy—but simply to illustrate the deeply rooted and intense fear cancer can bring out in many patients. J.R.'s story is not rare, and given the choice, many patients prefer frequent examination just for the sake of hearing and rehearing the magic words that declare the absence of cancer. Most are embarrassed to admit it or don't want to impose on their doctor. J.R. was merely more vocal than most about his desires and more assertive in his demands. I believe it is accurate to say that I have never had a patient complain about an overly conscientious follow-up schedule.

My rule of thumb has always been if a patient needs to be seen more frequently, so be it. I have always told patients not to smolder with anxiety and insecurity if they experience something disturbing in the posttreatment period, and rather than waiting one or two months for the routine checkup, they should call to arrange to be seen sooner. If nothing else, it's good psychotherapy for them to know it's the norm to be scared. Obviously, this tends to clutter the waiting list in a surgeon's practice, but such a problem should be accepted as part of the deal upon entering oncology.

This availability serves to illustrate one of the differences between cancer surgery and other surgical subspecialties. I remember operating on a family member of a cardiac surgeon friend of mine. He witnessed the whole process while supporting his loved one. Unfortunately, the outcome was not good, and the cancer eventually won. My colleague witnessed me spending long periods comforting and helping the patient die. My friend later said to me, "Your world is so different than mine. I operate on patients, and most of the time they get better, and when they don't, they die, usually without the prolonged misery. To go through that repeatedly must be really exhausting, and your time commitment is unbelievable." I thought about the truth of that statement, and had to remind myself that the technical part of taking care of cancer patients should be but a small part of the picture—and as I said earlier in this book, the emotional rewards come from exactly what my friend was talking about. At the risk of suggesting that there is a neurotic component involved, this fact almost certainly to some degree relates to the cancer physician's own needs.

The fears of these patients are both simple and complex, and they extend from low grade to paralytic. Whether cured or not, the cancer victim often thinks of the darkness of night as a dreaded foe. The loneliness of the night catalyzes fear—and the night, different from the day, can be a miserable time. Worries about financial matters, family, dignity, pain, deformity, dependency on others, being abandoned and alone, loss of autonomy, and obviously death itself are all virtual shadows that go bump in the night. These are deep and dark fears with the power to invade dreams and even in a subconscious way drag the spirit down so that, upon awakening, the dominant companion is anxiety rather than optimism. On a number of occasions, I have been deluged with a patient's morbid description of sleepless nights in which everything from cellular growth to blood flow through their vessels are thought to have been felt or imagined. Much like the cardiac neurotic who lies in bed and feels and listens to every nuance of the heartbeat, the cancer patient's exquisite sense of body can be terrifying, and no matter how illogical or bizarre their fears, the physician must attentively listen and reassure. Never should these fears be minimized, and above all, humor should never be used to deflect concern. A serious attentiveness with eye contact are noticed and appreciated, while glibness and/or a distracted presence are resented.

A fairly common event for posttreatment cancer patients is to experience nightmares, most of which center around death-related experiences that, by the time of awakening, have dragged them down into an amorphous inferno of pessimism. Self-confidence has often been compromised or even shattered, and not infrequently, these patients are overwrought with anxiety. I try to preempt such an occurrence by telling patients that this might occur, and if it does, they should call my office. An earlier than scheduled office visit and the reassurance that their experience was a psychic boom—nothing more, nothing less—can do wonders. I have had discussions with other cancer physicians who responded to my depiction of such things with surprise, saying that they do not hear such things from patients. I submit to the reader that the reason for this is evident—their patients apparently don't feel invited to delve into such subliminal matters. Furthermore, I believe it to be self-delusional and naive for these physicians to think that their patients don't have similar fears.

Almost all cancer patients become much more aware of their bodies, and they often apply amateurish physical examination techniques that lead to the discovery of insignificant lumps and bumps, most of which have been there all along and usually have been noticed by their doctors. Whether the fear is more physical—a lump or a redness previously unnoticed, an odd symptom—or merely the aftermath of a bad dream, the most efficient way to overcome it is to invite the patient in for a quick check and certification of their disease-free state. The classic example of this is that emotional nemesis for women—the discovery of a breast lump. Even though eight of ten such lumps are ultimately found to be benign, the staccato of escaping subliminal fears that follow this revelation can become an emotional stampede. In any of these patients—the discovery of a lump, or the occurrence of a nightmare—asking them to wait for the next scheduled appointment is insensitive and inhumane. Lest the reader think all patients react this way, it should be said that the majority of people are able to move on with their life with routine follow-up and reassurance, sometimes untroubled by anything other than mild but chronic fear. Even in the bravest of patients, however, terror can lurk just below the surface, and the alarm bells ring when unexplained symptoms or signs appear.

As I mentioned in describing the emotional anguish of J.R., many patients begin building anxiety in the days and even weeks leading up to their routine check, so by the time of the visit to the cancer physician, the patient is on edge and fearful. Because of this, during follow-up visits I always made it a practice to greet patient and family with real friendliness, but only briefly—keeping the preliminaries to a minimum and moving quickly to the relevant questions and the examination. That is what is foremost on the minds of these people, and an audible sigh of relief is not an uncommon response to the magical phrase—"all's clear." Even more impressively, tears of relief sometimes come at this juncture, during which an embarrassed patient and the physician are able to share a sublime emotional moment with the privacy afforded by their duality. That certainly was the case with J.R. and me.

After the "all's clear," and only after, time is allotted to catching up on family and other non-cancer-related matters that provide conversational material between people who have often become friends. The emotionally committed physician should neither discount nor underrate the dependence and affection that these patients often feel for the person who they believed has saved them. It can be hurtful for the patient if the physician is unwilling to spend at least a short time on personal matters. Cancer patients frequently feel vulnerable and don't suffer their doctor's personal slights well.

Time is the enemy common to all busy physicians. By now, it probably has occurred to the reader that all of this personalized attention and on-the-job psychotherapy takes a lot of time. The unscheduled intrusions, the need for reassurance time and time again, and other interactions all come at the expense of the physician's personal life as well as his other patients. Most people have had the frustrating experience of sitting and sometimes pacing for hours in a crowded waiting room, only to be greeted by an overbooked, behind-schedule doctor who is trying to catch up while trying to appear unrushed. I won't try to minimize the aggravation of this—my own family members have had the experience on a number of occasions. It happens too often, but on many occasions, the delays are unavoidable, and in the world of the cancer physician, the problem is a chronic one for all of the reasons that I have referred to in this section. Cancer patients often are easily and quickly reassured and take the allotted time only; however, there are many that demand more—both demonstrably and emotionally. They need to talk, and within reason, to deny them is callous. I readily admit to having kept many people waiting for long periods, but almost always, when they did get into the exam room, they were the focus of my attention, and within reason, got as much time and attention as they needed.

In reality, most cancer patients are extraordinarily understanding of the time issue with their physician, and are readily forgiving of delays. This is so because when their turn comes, they know they won't be rushed. Cancer patients share an unspoken commonality of fears and anxieties, and they respect the honesty of the physician's efforts to apportion enough time and emotional support to all patients, even if it means delay for others. Having said this, all oncologists have encountered patients who are almost impossible to satisfy. In an effort to be generous with time, the office waiting room can become bogged down, and this creates a real frustration for the physician. Knowing that multiple people are frustrated and sometimes angry adds to the burden already on the physician. It is inaccurate for patients to think the physician doesn't care about the time issue—just the opposite is usually true; therefore, when a physician walks in after major delay and appropriately starts the visit with a sincere apology, the patient should accept it and move forward.

In the early 1980s, I successfully operated on the elderly mother of a dear friend and colleague. The patient, A.R., was a wonderful human being who had been happily indulged throughout her life by a doting physician husband, and a very attentive son—also a physician. Probably because of the loneliness of her widowed state she insisted on coming to the office frequently, and on each occasion she took a huge amount of time, asking me questions about much of her health profile, most of which was unrelated to her cancer. She wasn't frightened, and was confident of cancer cure; she wanted to deal with other health-related issues. Mrs. R. had truly adopted me as her general doctor! Because of my affection for both her and her son, I was overly indulgent, and even instructed my staff to alter the office schedule on days when she was scheduled for a visit. Minutes often turned into an hour, and the waiting room was backed up accordingly. Her son was well aware of the situation, and he and I would share a smile when it came up. One day, Mrs. R. gave me the usual hug and kiss when I came into the exam room, and then admonished me, "This time, I don't want you to rush me like you usually do." I later shared this story with her son and he and I enjoyed a hardy laugh—respectful and loving—at the expense of an insatiably needy elderly lady who somehow thought that I had neglected her. We both understood that there was no need for him to apologize for his mother.

The take-home message of this section is that, as with raising children, in caring for cancer patients, the needs differ from one person to the next. Some require more attention, some less; if a physician does not have the flexibility to cater to this diverse emotional appetite, he or she should work in another part of medicine. This is in no way meant to diminish the contributions of my colleagues who work in specialties less emotionally demanding then oncology.

The fact that the cancer physician must function at a heightened emotional level, often in an atmosphere of sadness, fear, and suffering, is essential to the cautionary message of this book, and the aspiring cancer doctor must be comfortable in embracing the enormous responsibility and time commitment of caring for patients whose dependence, vulnerability, and psychological fragility all leap from the ordinary. The casual observer justifiably might wonder, "Why not just refer these patients to a psychiatrist or psychologist and be done with it? Why get so emotionally involved?" In fact, most sophisticated cancer teams do include psychiatric colleagues who frequently become involved with initial consultation and often repeated therapeutic sessions. However, their participation—even when effective—does not preclude the emotional involvement of other members of the team, whose emotional responsibilities are in no way mutually exclusive of those of the psycho-oncologist. Obviously, the administration of medication in the treatment of related depression is left to those who are schooled with this new pharmacopoeia.

Even before the maturation of modern-day psycho-oncology,[4] I consistently relied on the psychiatry community in my care of cancer patients. However, the recent evolution of this valuable subspecialty and the development of both the antidepressants and the antianxiety medications have made a huge difference in the care of cancer patients.

A patient's response to the psychiatry referral often depends on the method of presentation. When it's done without adequate explanation, many

patients think, "I have enough trouble now without trying to dig into my relationship with my parents." The public's perception of psychiatry as an analytical endeavor that involves "time on the couch" is outmoded and inaccurate, at
least as it pertains to cancer. Importantly, such traditional thinking cripples
the acceptance of modern methods. Sigmund Freud, the father of the analytic
method, died after a long and painful bout with oral cancer, for which there
was then, as there is now, little applicability of analytical principals. So it
should be made clear to patients that the contemporary psychiatry that applies
to the world of cancer medicine is built on the principles of situational help
for a specific situational problem—the cancer. Importantly, modern psycho-
oncology is action oriented, supportive, and fully utilizes liberal intervention
with the new generation of medications. I will come back to the theme of
psychiatric help later, but at this juncture, suffice it to say that the psycho-
oncologist is integral to achieving the contemporary standard of cancer care.

It is important that, even when a psychiatrist is involved in a patient's
care, the other members of the cancer team, especially the other oncologists—
whether they are surgical, radiation, or medical—should not think of their
role only as mechanical providers of that which is tangible. Not infrequently,
during the course of prolonged cancer treatment, an "alpha member" of the
team is identified or evolves in the mind of the patient. Depending on the
personalities involved, the patient may develop a more intense bond with
and depend more on one particular member of the team. Whenever I found
myself in that role, I viewed it as an important additional responsibility that
required my continued availability to the patient and family, despite the fact
that my phase of the treatment strategy—surgery—may have ended, and
the chemotherapy or radiation phase of the treatment was underway. In the
course of radiation or chemotherapy treatments, certain events and side effects can and do occur, and despite the reassurance of the treating team, the
patient sometimes feels the need for contact with that alpha person.

It goes without saying that if not handled carefully, such multilateral
counseling carries the potential for contradictions and confusion, both of
which can undermine the treating oncologist. If approached intelligently and
unselfishly, however, such aid can be invaluable for a patient and also serve to
fortify the confidence in the cancer team concept. Within the experiences of the
patient, psychological support is best delivered circumferentially, coming from
all members of the team. The patient's awareness of the interactive dialogue
between members of the cancer team—that is to say, the unit's functionality—
provides immeasurable reassurance when it is seen working smoothly.

Not infrequently, patients sense team dysfunction in which they doubt
the communication among its members is efficient. Whether accurate or not,
the perception of dysfunction in itself can be disconcerting to a patient.

· 5 ·

Hope

Hope springs eternal in the human breast: Man never is, but always to be blest.

—*Alexander Pope (1688–1744)*

The unwillingness of a cancer physician to contribute to the emotional equation between doctor and patient often stymies the latter's ability to develop real hope. The importance of hope in life's experiences can be seen in the Greek myth of Pandora. According to legend, Zeus gave Pandora, the first mortal woman, a box that she was forbidden to open. Within it were all human blessings and curses. Despite Zeus's admonition not to open the box, curiosity overcame Pandora's restraint—and open it she did. In a moment, all of the curses were released into the world, and all the blessings escaped and were lost, except one—hope. Without hope, mortals could not endure.

Too often in the past the belief that true hope is an important component in the healing of cancer's multiple depletions has been considered mere psychobabble or at best received only lip service in orthodox oncology circles. But in the practical world of cancer medicine, there is nothing psychologically more valuable to give than hope—as long as it is realistic and honest; hence, the distinction made between true and false hope. Better for the doctor to be noncommittal than to encourage false hope. The reader should be cautious not to equate curing of cancer's depletions with curing of the cancer itself, that is, hope doesn't necessarily apply to the latter.

As I will show in this writing, in the lexicon of cancer, hope must be redefined to include achievements other than cure. A rich and compelling analysis of this underrated human need is provided in Jerome Groopman's book, *The Anatomy of Hope*.[1] In this work, the author draws on numerous poignant anecdotes from his lifetime of practicing medical oncology. Importantly, he cogently argues that there is almost certainly a neurochemical basis for hope as a critical component in facing adversity. In seeking to define hope, he first separates it from optimism. Unlike blind optimism, "hope is rooted in unalloyed reality." It "acknowledges the significant obstacles and deep pitfalls" along the pathway. Groopman feels that there is no room for delusion in true hope. Positive thinking, while useful, does not alone produce hope. Rather, Groopman says, "Hope is the elevating feeling we experience when we see— in the mind's eye—a path to a better future."[2] As a means of underscoring these limitations, the well-known psycho-oncologist, Jimmie Holland, refers to "the tyranny of positive thinking."[3] I want to add to this line of thinking my belief that the trust generated by the physician-patient relationship is the most important catalyst that nourishes true hope. From the integrity of this relationship comes real trust, and from that, the patient's capacity for hope. When possible, however, it is appropriately within the purview of the cancer physician to help the patient find true hope. After all, the setting for this is ripe. To quote Sir Walter Scott, "Hope is brightest when it dawns from fears,"[4] and as I have pointed out, the cancer experience is universally frightening.

Significantly, the integrity to which I refer must be sacrosanct, and when it is time for the physician to be the bearer of bad news, there is no honest role for false hope. Elliptical answers represent a form of abandonment, and when the reality of the situation becomes known, the patient will often feel betrayed and angry. Groopman relates a moving story in which one of his medical on-cology preceptors allowed a certain cancer patient and her family to continue to believe in the possibility for cure, even though the malignancy had become unresponsive to drugs. When the young physician questioned the propriety of this, he was admonished that in some patients, ignorance is bliss. When the truth shortly became obvious, however, the patient's daughter scolded, "I guess you didn't think people like us are smart enough, or strong enough to handle the truth."[5]

In telling this story, Groopman's remorse and embarrassment are almost palpable as he concedes that by withholding the truth, he and his preceptor had abandoned the patient and left family members alienated and bitter. Ignorance obviously had not been blissful for this family, as the preceptor had believed. Most of us at some point have succumbed to the temptation to take the easy way out by not delivering bad news. In fairness to the story-teller, however, he was the junior man, and the patient was really under his teacher's care—to behave differently would have been very awkward. Even his complicity in the evasion, however, appropriately caused Doctor Groopman to feel guilty.

Evasion and avoidance of face-to-face confrontation with truth might be temporarily easier for the family and physician when dealing with a dying patient, and while such behavior may be well intended, its overall effect is usually harmful. In my experience, the negatives associated with this method outweigh what is temporarily gained. About ten years ago, a friend of mine called to ask my advice about his teenage niece who had just been diagnosed with an ominous sarcoma of the lung. I referred her to a noted oncologist in a major cancer center. The plan for chemotherapy and surgery was suggested and started. After initial encouragement, the tumor reappeared in the chest wall, and surgery was again employed, radiation therapy and further chemotherapy were given, but all to no avail. During the two weeks before her death the patient was hospitalized with complications secondary to the chemotherapy, and the cancer was obviously on a relentless path. In the final period, in which impending death was obvious to the cancer team, no one was allowed to talk to this young woman about death, and when one of the team members alluded to what might be happening, the patient herself interrupted and said that she didn't want to have a negative conversation. She added that anyone unwilling to continue fighting would not be welcomed in her room. Up to the actual death, the charade was played out, and in fact, the family boasted about her being "a real fighter." No member of the intimidated medical team had stepped up and required the patient and family to think realistically.

With everyone in denial, with the fantasy continuing, and with the hopeless battle raging, there were no comforting exchanges, and closure was not achieved. Instead, the last six weeks of this young woman's life were spent accompanied by the misery of nausea, vomiting, immune suppression, and other problems related to meaningless therapy. Essentially, any semblance of tranquility was absent in the frantic fight to the death. This is a classic case of allowing the patient and family to have false hope—similar to the story told by Groopman, but yet different in some respects. With his patient, there was actual reassurance, whereas in the story I just told, the physicians took the path of least resistance by allowing the patient and family to dictate the course of events. While both circumstances would illicit different opinions from different individuals, I believe that neither case was emotionally well handled.

I stated earlier in this section that trust in a physician—especially when discussing cancer—is integral to a patient's hope. To trust is to have faith and confidence not only in the integrity and unselfishness but especially the beneficence of the person in charge; bottom line: "Will my doctor do and advise what is best for me?" Periodically throughout this book, I mention the role of the cancer physician as a leader. In the world of oncology, the ability to find a balance between empathy and guidance throughout the cancer journey is the sine qua non of good leadership. The paradigm is straightforward: Good doctor/patient relations come out of honest and forthright dialogue that is based on realism rather than paternalistic avoidance of unpleasant news. Such a relationship begets trust of the physician, which in turn begets acceptance of the inevitable, as the patient is led to that place that Kathleen Dowling Singh refers to as the great mystery at the edge of life and death.[6]

The importance of the relationship between trust and hope can't be overstated, and because the two are inextricably linked, it is appropriate to discuss them in parallel. To point out the obvious, cancer patients obviously have serious trouble and extraordinary needs, and the process of dealing with them is made easier by a game plan that is succinct and understandable from start to finish and that is well communicated by a take-charge cancer physician in a compassionate and honest manner. Ideally, such a doctor guides the patient to a workable definition of hope, that is, what is achievable rather than what is desired. To paraphrase Peter Ubel, the more confident patients are in the truthfulness of the person running the show, the less vulnerable they are to distracting feelings, superstitions, and fears that motivate them to make bad choices.[7] People tend to accept anecdotes that draw them away from statistics and reality. It would seem that almost every cancer patient encounters someone along the way who had a relative or a friend with a similar problem and their "doctor did such and such," to paraphrase most unsolicited advice. As much as possible, physicians should present data clearly and in doing this, simplify choices. Most of all, even though the final decisions rest with the patient and family, the physician must stay in control of the dialogue.

Actually, all of the definitions of hope have one thing in common—they deal with the expectation of good that is yet to be; that is to say, with a perception of a future condition in which a desired goal will be achieved. Within these parameters, by building on trust and creditable dialogue, a physician can help a patient find closure in life and an acceptance of death, both of which add tranquility to the final stage of existence.

Too often, physicians misunderstand hope by thinking only in terms of cure or remission. This flawed concept is common in the ever-optimistic oncology community—surgical, radiation, and medical alike. Hope can also be for a good death; for mending of interpersonal bonds that are in disrepair; for resolution of one's own feelings about divinity and a life after death; and, yes, for comforting loved ones who will be left behind.

I have treated several patients with advanced cancer whose main interest was to live long enough to participate in major family events such as a birth or a wedding. I remember one patient we treated for a "hopeless" situation, inducing partial remission of the cancer that allowed a man to walk his daughter to the wedding alter. Four weeks afterward, he took his own life. On a number of occasions, I have witnessed Roman Catholics facing death with extreme fear and trepidation, only to achieve an obvious state of tranquility when a priest entered the room, intent on administering the last rites.[8] In another section of this book, I'll speak more on the passage from life to death, and in that context will elaborate on this quintessential Roman Catholic practice.

These various situations and motives—"a good death," the comfort of closure brought to relationships, attending a family function, dying in the good graces of one's creator, among other circumstances—reflect a redefinition of hope. Never mind what the medical team deems important, the patient is the author of the new standard, and it is the job of the physician to incorporate that into the dialogue of the relationship.

On a broader scale, perhaps hope resides in the realization of what our lives have been, or to utilize the thinking of the Roman philosopher, Seneca, how well one lives is more important than how long.[9] Doctors—especially oncologists with the best of intentions—too often fight the battle to excess, and in an effort to "do something," use up valuable end-of-life time and resources. Sherwin Nuland views this desperate behavior as reflective of our current society's refusal to admit the existence of death's power, and perhaps even death itself. He points out that in this high-tech biomedical era, when the tantalizing possibility of miraculous cures is dangled before patient and family, the temptation to see therapeutic hope is great, even in those situations when common sense would suggest otherwise.[10]

In her book, *The Grace in Dying*, Kathleen Dowling Singh, a person of deep spiritualism and an expert on death and dying, discusses the importance of exploring these very emotional subjects with patients. By doing this, the natural inclination to hold our mortality at bay can be overcome. Dowling Singh believes that such discussions reflect a maturing culture that has begun to more readily embrace death as a part of life. Such things as hospice care and death counseling have an overall effect of allowing the course of death to be less impeded.[11] While I agree, I can't help but be struck by the irony of this author's reference to a culture "maturing" by embracing what our forefathers understood and accepted readily; in truth, we are maturing by utilizing wisdom garnered from history. With this realization, we have come full circle by drawing back somewhat from a mind-set that modern technology and science have fostered—that of never giving up. It is important that the reader not misunderstand my motives for introducing these thoughts; my intention is certainly not to stymie the scientific search for adding time and quality to life. On the contrary, this has been one of the common denominators of my life's work. Instead, by exploring these thoughts, I am making a plea for realism in dealing with the inexorability of death.

In deciding how much treatment is enough, the cancer physician must repeatedly address the question of what is in the best interest of the patient. Even if what is done turns out to be the wrong strategy, if the motive was in quest of the patient's benefit, it is morally defensible. This sounds simplistic, but in fact, pride, vanity, and other unresolved or perhaps even unrecognized psychic forces within a physician can complicate a patient's life and death. Physicians, like other talented and intelligent people, are not immune to the insecurity that seeks reassurance of their abilities, and whether realized or not, part of their self-image depends on success and failure in patient care. Additionally, many physicians are extraordinarily competitive, and the instinct to fight on can be strong. Some oncologists seem to feel obligated to explore every avenue of treatment, no matter how unlikely the benefit. Whether we like it or not, aside from this being void of beneficence, it is financially an unsupportable strategy.

In a yet-to-be-published study conducted at the U.S. Centers for Disease Control and Prevention,[12] the investigators found that the cost of treating cancer in the United States nearly doubled over the past two decades, a fact that was largely due to the increasing number of cancer patients. The seriousness of this situation is real: The projected numbers future cases were developed on a realistic model that illustrates that cancer continues to exact a major toll on the nation. In 2005, for example, almost 1.5 million new cases of cancer were diagnosed in the United States, and almost half of them died of their disease. Cancer has recently surpassed heart disease as the leading cause of death among Americans under age 85, even though prevention efforts, early detection, and better treatments have been responsible for the total number of cancer deaths per 100,000 gradually declining about 1 percent per year since 1999.[13] However, medicine is making relatively more progress in lowering the mortality secondary to heart disease. The paradigm is clear for most cancers, risk rises with age, and the U.S. population over age 65 is growing rapidly.[14] Accordingly, the annual number of new cancer cases is expected to grow, potentially doubling by 2050.[15]

Additionally, successful treatment is responsible for more people living with or having been cured of cancer. This is obviously good; however, the overall associated cost—that reflected in the quoted CDC study—is on a collision course with the costs of unrealistic cancer treatment in which there is little or no benefit. Over the last thirty years, the number of cancer cases covered by Medicare has increased substantially; in fact, oncology currently accounts for 40 percent of Medicare's overall drug costs.[16] Undoubtedly, the new cancer-related drugs now in phase III trials will eventually accentuate this expense, but the basis of the increasing expense will continue to be the number of patients. We must question a system that is set up to encourage the overuse of treatments with little to no expectation of benefit rather than dealing realistically with death by the incorporation of palliative measures. By the use of therapy that is unlikely to be effective, oncologists actually do a disservice to the system by depleting patient and industry resources. In particular, they harm patients by generating false hope.

So as to take this out of the realm of speculation, I point to a study recently reported in the Annals of Internal Medicine that used patients from California and Massachusetts as a study cohort.[17] All were sixty-five and older and had died as a result of their cancer. In over 20 percent of the study group, chemotherapy had been administered within three months prior to their death, and significantly, the cancer's responsiveness to chemotherapy did not seem to influence whether dying patients received chemotherapy at the end of life. Use of chemotherapeutic agents was similar for patients with breast, colon, and ovarian malignancies and even for those with cancers that are generally considered unresponsive to chemotherapy, such as melanomas and those of the pancreas, liver, and kidney.[18] Circumstantial data from another study showed that 20 percent of the Medicare cancer patients with metastasis who were analyzed had been started on a new chemotherapy regimen within two weeks of death.[19] The implications of this are far-reaching and profound, and among cynics surely suggest monetary motives. One is left to speculate how this data would differ in a population of uninsured patients. In evaluating what seems like a system's error, the obvious question is that if there are incentives for oncologists to try more treatment despite minimal odds for success, why can't the reverse be implemented? Why can't there be disincentives to go for that long shot?

A cascade of aggressive care often results from a poorly planned entrance into what I refer to as the descending stairway of managing refractory and/or advanced cancer. Above all else, physicians must avoid deception when traveling in this zone, and when dealing with these patients, rather than forgoing hope, often it is better to redefine it. I think of this as guidance of patient and family expectations, and it seems to be a responsibility frequently handled badly. Early in the journey down this virtual stairway, the physician must discuss a realistic prognosis with the patient, because when the final decline is unanticipated, the "cascade" begins and moves forward with a rapid staccato of events, many of which represent care of diminishing value that promotes physical, psychological, and spiritual suffering that can leave a family overwhelmed and ultimately devastated financially. It is entirely appropriate to demonize this cascade as a phenomenon that, once started, seems to acquire independent momentum—intensive care, organ failure and multiple machines, increasing sedation, patient confusion, and the disorientation that is unofficially known as ICU psychosis—like a tumbleweed in a desert wind. By this time, the patient is often unable to make rational and unemotional decisions and choices. At a minimum, patient and family spirits have gone down while the costs have gone up, and a thoughtful person should ask if the duration of useful life has actually been increased.

It has been said that like fire and water, modern technology can be a wonderful servant, but a point is reached when it becomes a bad master. I think of this state as fantasy gone berserk, in which a theorized "technotopia" has actually become "dystopia." So as it pertains to my earlier-used phrase—the descending stairway of advancing cancer—my plea is for an early reality check, since the treatment decisions made near the end are prone to propel a dying person in a senseless direction. With that said, it is important to concede the need for certain palliative surgical techniques that are humanely applicable to those approaching death. For example, in certain selective circumstances, operations such as a gastrostomy, a colostomy, a tracheostomy, or a rhizotomy can diminish the misery of intestinal, airway, and neurological compromises.

The reader might think that my deviation has resulted from distraction—not so. This particular discussion started with the importance of cancer patients being able to find hope in their plight; and by intentionally steering the discussion to the misallocation of effort and resources in the advanced cancer patient, I seek to emphasize my earlier premise that only through a trusting relationship is a patient able to completely rely on a physician's unselfish guidance in making practical choices at the end of life. In this journey to one's end, hope is ideally redefined with the help of a trusted physician who is able to strike a balance between empathy and functionality. Critical to all of this is the principle that the patient and the family—not the physician or the third-party payers—should actually dictate that redefinition.

Finally, there is that hope that is based on optimistic data—the prognosis is good. I refer to this as the hope derived from realistic expectations. After all, people with many types of cancer are surviving longer following their diagnosis than at any time in the past. The financial issues cited in previous paragraphs aside, the overall five-year relative survival rate for all cancers combined is now 64 percent, and an estimated 9.8 million Americans are living with a cancer history.[20] Many cancers are cured 90 percent of the time. Even in hopeful situations, however, the treatment enactment can be prolonged and draining—daily radiation treatments for up to two months, simultaneous chemotherapy, and in many cases surgery at some point in the sequence, perhaps in the beginning, perhaps at the end. During this marathon of misery euphemistically referred to as the cancer treatment plan, physical discomfort, the inability to sleep despite exhaustion, discouragement, and depression can come together to form an anchor that must be dragged almost by shear force of will. I have had many patients tell me that the proverbial "light at the end of the tunnel"—the thought of the end of treatment and a new start were essential to their endurance. I mentioned earlier in this section that all definitions of hope included the expectation of good that is yet to be, a perception of a future condition in which a desired goal will be achieved. Finishing the marathon is more the norm than the exception—somehow most of these patients manage to see it through. What is surprising, however, is that a number of patients do more than endure. They come to view the experience as a turning point in their lives in which they reevaluate former lifestyles, relationships, work habits, goals, and the general value system in which they have previously functioned. While preparing to write this book, I interviewed a number of patients in some detail about this subject, and many tell of finding new levels of love and companionship with spouse and children not previously experienced. Many found a new level of value to life itself, often exercising the option to stop and smell the roses; and even more alluring to these individuals after the self-analysis was the desire to "pay back" and make a contribution to the improvement of the human condition—and in doing this, find more meaning in life.

· 6 ·

Finding New Purpose after
Enduring the Cancer Olympics

$\mathcal{O}$f all of the rewards that I have received from treating cancer patients, the most gratifying are those gained from productive posttreatment life changes made by cancer patients who have endured the "Cancer Olympics."[1] Many stories come to mind in this regard, but three that stand out are briefly depicted below. A summary of each story is important to the theme of this section, and I ask the reader's patience with my self-indulgence in resurrecting these happy memories.

During the 1980s, when I was a member of the Head and Neck Surgical team at Memorial Sloan-Kettering Cancer Center in New York City, a middle-age man (B.K.) was referred to me for a base of skull cancer of substantial proportions, and the treatment part of the strategy involved a prolonged course of radiation therapy, which was of course administered by a radiation oncology colleague. I served mostly as the quarterback—diagnosis, workup, and the appropriate referral. The patient was part of the leadership—actually head of one of the three divisions of one of the largest and most successful corporations in the world. For him to be at that level at that age was remarkable, and he was on track to eventually head this giant corporation. In all respects, he was a strong and enduring patient, bubbling over with drive and a positive attitude, but pleasantly free of arrogance—feeling no self-pity, and committed entirely to winning the war in which he found himself. That did happen, and afterward, he took stock of his previous immersion in the corporate jungle, decided on other outlets for his energy, and retired. He became the president of a nonprofit foundation devoted to a national effort to link up cancer patients with other individuals from around the country who had similar cancers. This pro-bono job occupied much of his time, during which he raised money and provided leadership for this important organization for a number of years. Recently, my wife and I joined him and his wife for dinner in celebration of his twenty-fifth year of freedom from cancer, and during the course of the evening, he actually said to me that in a perverse sort of way, undergoing the cancer experience was one of the most positive events of his life. It had forced him to take stock and reevaluate, and the adjustments and actions that resulted were substantially more fulfilling and gratifying than his previous activities. The fact that he and his family savored the afterglow of cure together and enhanced their relationships was an added bonus.

A patient (M.B.) that I treated at the Georgetown Medical Center in Washington, D.C. during the 1990s was thirty-four years old at the time of his operation for thyroid cancer. Although moderate in size, his cancer was a favorable variety, and he has gone on to live a healthy life after returning to his former employment. In addition, he created a national thyroid support group that offered an online support network, and put on a yearly conference—each year located in a different part of the country—that was designed for thyroid cancer patients. Essentially, this is an academic program for survivors, and it is attended by a surprisingly diverse sample of patients from around the country. C.G. raises the money to run this entire program, including the yearly conferences. At the conferences, the faculty consists of guest speakers—endocrinologists, nuclear medicine specialist, surgeons, and scientists whose research relates to thyroid cancer, all of whom donate their time. I spoke at one of the meetings, and I must say, the audience was well prepared with intelligent questions, and everyone was full of curiosity about the medical standards concerning this disease. The day that I lectured to the group stands out in my memory because the whole experience literally swelled me with pride for my patient, who had seen light at the end of the tunnel and who had emerged from it with renewed gusto and creativity. In his way, he truly was helping to improve the human condition.

Another of my Memorial Sloan-Kettering patients that I operated on in the 1980s was a young superstar from one of the iconic financial institutions of New York City. J.C. had been educated in economics, and in her late twenties was well on her way to a stellar career on Wall Street. Fortunately, I was able to successfully operate on an aggressive malignancy of her soft palate. Her attitude was upbeat and combative toward the cancer, and during this very stressful time, she proved what an outstanding young person she was. She was so affected by the whole cancer experience that she quit her job, went back to undergraduate school to get the prerequisites for entry into medical school, and then went on to attend Johns Hopkins School of Medicine in Baltimore. She stayed at Hopkins to complete a residency in emergency medicine. Somewhere along the way, she married, had a couple of kids, and even found time to train for and run a marathon. For years, I received Christmas cards from her—each was a heartwarming reward.

Not infrequently, cancer survivors volunteer to work in or around cancer treatment programs at cancer centers. On many occasions, I employed former patients to counsel those who had the same tumor for which they had been successfully treated. Few actions are more useful to a frightened patient than to spend time with a functional person who has previously faced the same problem—same cancer—same treatment—same fears—even the same medical team. Additionally, I have always attempted to match people with similar profiles and life experiences, thus enhancing the ease with which the patient identifies with the volunteer. Importantly, the volunteer is encouraged to be honest and not to mitigate the misery factor with an unrealistically rosy depiction of what they are facing. This "tough love" counseling is far more creditable then a disingenuous avoidance of unpleasant subjects that is soon to be encountered during treatment. There is little need for a cheerleader at this point. This concept of matching has proven valuable and rewarding to patient and volunteer alike. The construction worker might have different anxieties than a college professor, and thus the matching of each with an appropriate counterpart usually proves to be more productive.

One of the most heart-wrenching memories of my career involved the pairing of two young career women—both in their early forties—each of whom had tongue cancer. B.C. was a television reporter for a prominent local channel in a major city. I treated her for tongue cancer with surgical resection and reconstruction that was followed with radiation therapy. All indications favored a cure, and for a year she worked diligently with a speech therapist, all the while determined to regain the ability to articulate speech to a level that would allow her to resume her career in front of the television camera. Initially, I doubted that this was possible, but her determination and hard work happily overcame all else while she scoffed at my skepticism. In the meantime, I had seen another young woman—a businesswoman—with a similar problem who required identical management. Although B.C. was only one year out of treatment, we were optimistic for cure; therefore, I introduced her to the new patient, E.C. They quickly found commonality in their affliction, and became fast friends. B.C. even used E.C. to make a television documentary on oral cancer, using interviews with the patient and her doctors, discussing the disease and its treatment. Importantly, the articulation of the commentator—B.C.—was precise, and in a powerful closing sentence to the documentary, she said that this subject was of great personal interest to her because she too had been a victim of tongue cancer. That chapter of the story is the happy and gratifying part; unfortunately, the following year, B.C. developed lung metastasis and died, and the year following that, E.C.

suffered the same fate. These young women had found new purpose in life, although ultimately the demon that is cancer prevailed in both. The love and support shared by them came from careful matching in a useful volunteer program.

A number of high-profile individuals who have undergone cancer treatment have become active in public service as a result of their disease. Prominent examples of cancer victims who have used their star status for important public announcements and awareness messages include Lance Armstrong, who has devoted much energy and time to the promoting public awareness of the disease of testicular cancer. The prominent actor Jack Klugman, a survivor of laryngeal cancer, was very active in the antismoking campaign associated with that disease. During the last part of his life, the actor Yul Brynner was an avid antismoking campaigner. He had been a "chain smoker" for years, and, not surprisingly, died of lung cancer. At another point in this book, I speak of two women, Ambassador Shirley Temple Black and First Lady Betty Ford, who helped bring the subject of breast cancer out of the shadows of shame by going public with their own personal and thankfully successfully struggles with this disease. Their efforts were groundbreaking and have undoubtedly saved countless lives over the years since. Most recently, film icon Michael Douglas, himself a cancer survivor, has lent his support to a public service organization, the Cancer Alliance. These are but a few celebrities who have found purpose and meaning in a life after cancer. The list is much longer, and the exclusion of others is not meant to diminish the importance of their service.

Many patients of financial means find gratification by making monetary gifts or even by active fund-raising on behalf of cancer-related projects, research and otherwise. The various cancer programs require large sums of money to function. The national government is important to this endeavor, but that which comes out of the private sector is essential also, and much of that results from activities of former cancer patients.

I could refer to many patients who have changed their lives radically after the "Cancer Olympics" and many others who went back to their previous lives; in both categories, it's safe to say that they were all emotionally changed by the experience. Importantly, many patients discover that a meaningful life after cancer is possible. To paraphrase what I previously said, the period for getting over the experience is endless—and even when cured, the memory lurks just below the surface. Fortunately, however, the stage of acute anxiety diminishes rapidly, and once the person learns to live with the issue, a varying degree of emotional security usually follows. With the passage of time, people are usually better able to reengage in productive life.

· 7 ·

Changing Times, Changing Methods, Unchanging Mission

$\mathscr{F}$ollowing military service in the War Between the States, my great-grandfather, Samuel Compton (pictured in chapter 1), practiced medicine for twenty-five years in a small Louisiana town. During this time, he would leave home in a horse-drawn buggy to make house calls—often staying away for weeks at a time. I think of Doctor Compton whenever I look at the wonderful painting, *Doctor on the Bayou* (p. 40) by the well-known Louisiana artist, George Rodriguez, the artist depicts a country doctor of that era. Such men were paid with a combination of respect, love, gratitude, farm products, and every so often, money, which was in very short supply in the South after the Civil War. In reality, aside from draining abscesses, reducing fractures, doing amputations, and delivering babies, my great-grandfather probably had little tangible impact on his patients' various conditions, despite the fact that he was a well-educated and dedicated public servant. He undoubtedly administered "remedies" such as mustard plaster, herbs, potions, and purgatives; however, his real value was probably his presence. Thankfully, bloodletting had largely gone out of favor by the mid-nineteenth century, so I doubt if he was guilty of that. Truth be known, it is likely that "nature," that is to say, the immune systems of his patients, did most of the work in making patients better. In point of fact, Doctor Compton's house calls and many of his methods probably accomplished little, compared to the work of a contemporary doctor. Today, an emergency room team or a phoned-in antibiotic prescription quickly accomplishes more than my hardworking ancestor could have ever imagined. Compared to the physicians of yore, we labor in a medical utopia.

Given their extraordinary technological and scientific limitations, what is it then that my great-grandfather and other doctors of that era actually did—what was their role in helping the sick and injured? Surely, they had worth and

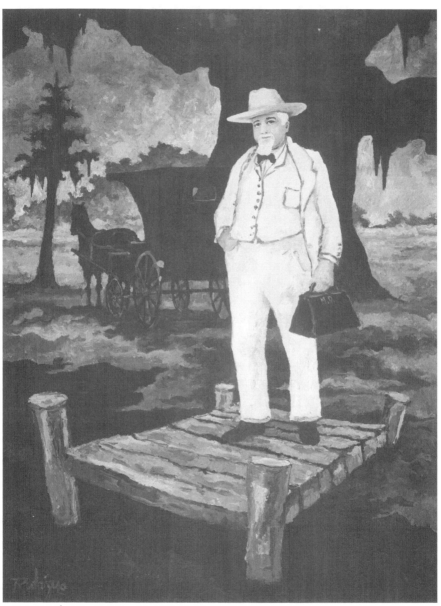

Doctor on the Bayou *by George Rodriguez. With the permission of the artist.*

value; they and other doctors before them were sought out and relied upon. After all, the profession has, since before Hippocrates, held a special place of reverence in most societies. To a great degree, I believe the answer relates to that essential action referred to in medical lingo as "the laying on of hands": they touched and they comforted. Without a doubt there was more, some of which was tangible, but in general it was the psychological connection between patient and doctor, something that I suspect has medicinal value.

Doctor Compton's story is obviously of genealogic interest to me, but that aside, I tell it because I suspect the personal connection between patient and doctor in those days was generally more intense than today, and furthermore the physician's dedication and concern helped to build a stronger bond, the value of which cannot be quantified. It's my belief that even though intangible, these human connections can and ought to be perpetuated in contemporary medical practice. Idealism and altruism, some of which are no more than romantic exaggerations, were certainly part of the mystique of the past, but in fairness to the physicians of today, patients and their families of less modern times had lower expectations. The public took for granted that doctors had many limitations, and importantly the patients and families of yore generally accepted most adversity and even medical failure much more readily than today. Illness and even death were considered but part of the life experience. While not scorned, death itself was accepted more readily than today, and most people of past times viewed it more philosophically.

Thomas Jefferson and John Adams died on the same day in 1826. During the twelve years that preceded their deaths, these iconic marvels enriched history with a treasure trove of correspondence between them, most of which has been preserved. In one notable letter, Jefferson bravely grappled with the issue of death—in a sense utilizing Darwinian logic—"There is a ripeness of time for death, regarding others as well as ourselves. When it is reasonable we should drop off, and make room for another growth. When we live our generation out, we should not wish to encroach on another."[1] A very thoughtful friend of mine likened life to standing in line for admission into some event; eventually, you get to the front of the line, and it's your time to step into the next realm.

It also should be pointed out that in these medically rudimentary times of the Founding Fathers and even in the later times of Doctor Compton, religion and faith were much more influential than they are today. Certain revered scholars such as Benjamin Franklin, Thomas Jefferson, and others, were thought to be deists,[2] who, while believing in God as a creator, thought "him" to be uninvolved with day to day life. Generally, however, the United States of America was founded and developed and the early Republic was led by people who believed God to be omnipresent, and involved in all things.

That attitude, for example was demonstrated vividly during the War between the States, in which General William Sherman and President Abraham Lincoln called on God for the success of the Union forces, and in the end, gave credit for victory to divine forces. Meanwhile my great-grandfather's bosses in the Army of Northern Virginia, General Robert E. Lee and General "Stonewall" Jackson were convinced of God's support and assistance for the Southern Confederacy. The point is that faith in those times was profound and was reflected in sayings like "It was God's will," "God had a purpose," or "God took them for a higher purpose," all of which were helpful and perhaps essential to personal perseverance after the frequent failures of medical science.

What choice did people have but to be accepting? Whether accomplished with anger or with divinely inspired equanimity, acceptance was the bottom line. One hundred fifty years ago, the profession was virtually helpless in combating most of what ailed people—yellow fever, smallpox, cholera, typhus, diphtheria, poliomyelitis, tetanus—the list is long. A wound, when infected was always life threatening, as were most internal problems like appendicitis, or even gall bladder disease. Children died from ear infections, measles, mumps, croup, and pneumonia. Even tonsillitis was a very serious problem that had a definable mortality rate. Tuberculosis (then referred to as consumption) usually ended fatally. Surgeons failed to cure even the simpler forms of cancer, and they had not even dreamt of attacking appendicitis and gall bladder disease. President George Washington died an agonizing death of asphyxiation, which probably resulted from a condition now called acute epiglottis in which certain bacteria cause the throat to swell and obstruct the airway. Today, the combination of steroids and antibiotics administered in an emergency room solves that problem within hours. President Ulysses Grant died of a tongue cancer that today probably would be cured with a combination of radiation and chemotherapy. The daughter of President John Adams died of a breast cancer that today would have been easily managed. The only death among the crew of the Lewis and Clark coast-to-coast expedition between 1802 and 1805 probably resulted from acute appendicitis and rupture[3]—a scenario that is today almost totally avoidable. As late as the early twentieth century, the young son of President Calvin Coolidge died from sepsis that developed from a simple blister on his foot; a phoned-in prescription of an antibiotic would today do the job. The list goes on and on. Therapeutic failures of that time reflected a dominance of disease over science. From a medical point of view, no matter how fictionally alluring that bygone time, those were not "the good old days."

Prior to modern-day therapeutic medical care, disease provided a moving platform, up and down, on which doctors were little more than passengers administering solace, soothing, and comfort, and in an attempt

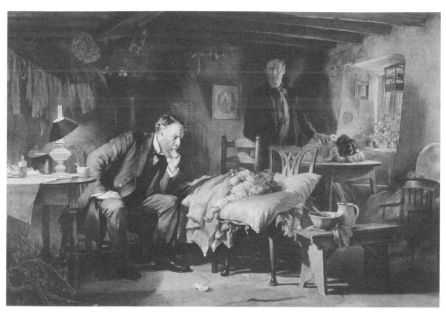

The Doctor *by Sir Luke Fildes (1891). Courtesy of the Dettrick Medical History, Case Western Reserve University.*

to do something—anything—probably often did harm. If one looks at the practices of my great-grandfather's time, what physicians did can seem absurd. In truth, their impotence reflects almost total ignorance of the etiology (disease cause) and pathogenesis (mechanism) of disease; thus the treatment was often targeted incorrectly, and more often than not, even if the disease had been understood, curative remedies were generally unavailable. Shown above is the famous painting from 1891 by Sir Luke Fildes, entitled *The Doctor*, that depicts the touching scene of a dying child, grieving parents, and a contemplative doctor at the child's side, probably having done as much as was possible, and only hoping—perhaps praying—for the best. This scene is visually a moving representation of what I have attempted to say in this section. Doctors of a different era had a limited knowledge and therapeutic ability, but the emotional bond between them and those who they served was often profound. I believe that we are still capable of this, and more.

In the time of Hippocrates, the average life expectancy was about twenty-five years. Though biomedical science has vastly increased that span of years, the maximum time of life has not changed in verifiable, recorded history. It would seem that even if one avoids pitfalls such as infectious disease, cancer, and cardiovascular disease, body parts still wear out within a finite time period.

To borrow once more from the rich trove of the Founding Fathers' wisdom, I point to a humorous but poignantly written letter from Thomas Jefferson at age seventy-one to the seventy-eight-year-old John Adams in which the former refers to their bodies as machines that "have been running seventy or eighty years, and we must expect that, worn as they are, here a pivot, there a wheel, now a pinion, next a spring will be giving way; and however we may tinker them up for a while, all will at length surcease motion."[4] To paraphrase Sherwin Nuland, all of the triumphs that we have achieved over pathology, no matter how ringing the victory, add up to only a reprieve from the inevitable end.

Because of biotechnological successes in thwarting that which once killed early in life, what kills us today has changed from the time of Doctor Compton's practice or even later, at the time of Fildes's painting. In those times, the infectious diseases that I mentioned decimated entire cultures, long before the killers of today—cardiovascular and lung disease, dementia, cancer, and even trauma—had a chance to take their grizzly toll. By 1900, the average life expectancy in the United States was forty-one; and by 2000, it had risen to seventy-seven years—amazingly, having doubled in only a century. The relatively short period during which medical science has evolved to preventing and curing disease is a testimony to the exponential growth of our knowledge; doctors are probably no smarter than before, only more educated. As a prelude to much that lies ahead in this book, it should be noted that the process of increasing life's average length, while wonderful, has created stupendous bioethical and sociological issues related to population excess, aging, quality of life and death, social and family responsibilities, and the physician's role as a healer and potentially as a taker of life.

Having pointed out some of the compelling differences between "then and now," and having ventured to make the case that doctor-patient relationships were more spiritual "then"—not religious, mind you, but more transcendental—than "now," the reader might pose the practical question—*So what?* Except for providing bedtime reading, how does all of this pertain to the current times in which we live and work? Addressing that question is, in fact, part of the practical basis for this book—I believe that a better transcendental connection between the profession and the lay public is still achievable. After all, why should contemporary science and human connection be mutually exclusive? Both physicians and patients have room for improvement in this realm.

It is worrisome that the image of today's medical profession seems different from what probably existed in times past. In fact, the increasing schism that seems to be developing in America between the profession and the lay public is an ominous trend. In dynamic social change, certain lines once broached are hard to return to. It is intuitive to me that the interest of the country is better served by doctors and patients staying in contact with each other, and it is my hope that this book will help to promote that.

Regarding the societal disconnect between doctors and patients, despite the less-than-ideal current relationship between them, I believe most people still possess a reservoir of goodwill and idealism regarding physicians. And I can vouch for the fact that most doctors still retain much of their idealism about patient care. Somehow, both the public and the profession have allowed a complex health care system with a tedious bureaucratic and corporate slant to come between them. Stopping this atrophy of mutual respect and goodwill is a goal worthy of everyone's attention. By making it clear that what is bad for doctors is usually ultimately bad for patients, we must try to bridge the two camps. It's far too simplistic, however, to only fault corporate America for doing what they do in the corporate way or the bureaucracy of governmental methods. Solutions do not lie in a "them against us" mentality, no matter how expedient it seems. That being said, corporate governance should take heed to keep in mind that individuals—physicians and patients alike—dislike being controlled from a boardroom; and the deeper the resentment, the more troubled the system and the more problematic the future. Somehow, all factions of this equation must seek the blend that will foster the salvation of what has served us so well in the past.

It is my opinion that the system's problems are complicated, but the solution to the schism involves the readjusting of the physician-patient relationship, rather than the relationship with corporate or government structure. I believe physicians can achieve true value in their interactions with patients only by taking the moral high ground. To use Edmund Pellegrino's wording, this level is achieved by acting not on the basis of what external forces do to the profession, but on the basis of what those forces do to those served by the profession.[5] I believe, as do many others, that the idealism of the physician-patient transcendent relationship should be the basis of the practice of medicine. Importantly, in our search for this level of idealism, many of the standards established in the Oath of Hippocrates, when modified for contemporary society, are part of the credo intuitively utilized by the vast majority of today's physicians. Even though not always required to recite or even know what is in the oath, doctors ought to realize that the words within retain their goodness of intent.

The fact that doctors don't always live up to patients' expectations usually relates to one of three factors: first, a failure of communication; second, a lack of patient realism, that is, failure to accept the fact that things don't always go according to plan; and, third, a lack of physician competence. At least as it pertains to oncology, the third of these is less frequently encountered than one might expect. The oncologists of today are better trained and just as dedicated as those of any other time. The other two factors—a lack of physician-patient communication and a lack of patient realism are often related, the latter being a result of the former. More will be said about the very important subject of communication later in this writing.

To say "times have changed" is more than an enormous understatement—it's a perversion of reality; and at a minimum, it is a stretch to compare the society and people of the past to those of today. It is essential, therefore, to understand that for better or worse, both patients and physicians reflect the new world. Wishing for the idealized version of what society and medicine used to be like, while it may be alluring (and is usually inaccurate), does not serve us well. In fact, I believe such a mind-set makes us less adaptable to the realities of the present. So, it is unrealistic to wish for contemporary physicians to behave like those portrayed in the past. Doctors are real, living, and breathing products of this era, and the public should be reminded that among their characteristics are the capacity for achievement as well as lethargy, success as well as failure, gentleness as well as rudeness, compassion as well as insensitivity, generosity as well as selfishness, stellar morals as well as moral judgmental lapses, mistakes, avarice, personality problems, and so on. Simply put, doctors are very much human. However, despite the many conflicting forces that have altered daily life, their mission has not changed, and many of the fundamental principles and ideals that have guided doctors in the past are worthy of perpetuation. Extraordinary social and scientific advances have influenced how medicine is practiced, but the moral and ethical values and codes of the past are generally adaptable to current times. That is to say, modernization and perpetuation of high-minded ethics are not mutually exclusive. The vast majority of today's physicians are, in fact, good and well-meaning public servants who intuitively behave in a moral and professional manner. As a result, they are in sync with the idealism of most of the original mission statement of the Hippocratic Oath. As the system is stressed, and even if the social atmosphere deteriorates further, we must continually monitor ourselves and reaffirm our ideals. In my role as an academic surgeon, I have continually interacted with the youth of the profession—medical students, interns, residents, those in fellowship training—and as a result of this exposure, I can speak with some authority about that generation of American doctors who easily equal the best of their counterparts in the nonmedical world.

While it may be fashionable to criticize the profession these days, the public should consider the legal climate as well as all of the tedious bureaucratic and administrative details with which the modern doctor must cope. When added to the enormous responsibilities of caring for the sick, there should be little wonder that there is considerable stress and unhappiness in the system. Even under these circumstances, however, most doctors are still highly motivated and are driven by ideals rather than greed, and most consistently try to do what is right for the patient rather than what is expedient. That said, it is only fair to concede that there are those in the universe of doctors not endowed with these qualities, and their actions serve to affirm my earlier statement that doctors are very much human. Greed and other selfish instincts disguised as necessities for self-preservation are seductive companions, and physicians committed only to self-interests should be condemned as sources of embarrassment to the vast majority who are not. The lay public should compartmentalize their contempt for this former group, and continue to think in a positive light of the profession as a whole.

Seeking Functionality within
a Moral Framework

Wrong is always wrong, even though everyone is doing it;
right is always right, even though no one is doing it.

—*Unknown Author*

As it pertains to the broad issue of physician behavior in the practice of medicine, it is both fair and appropriate to question whether medicine represents a higher calling, and to ask, if it does, isn't it logical that doctors should be held to a higher standard of morality than others in society? To answer these questions, we should first look at the medical world as it currently functions.

The eminent Georgetown University scholar Professor Edmund Pellegrino has said that practicing medicine in today's social climate is challenging and often demoralizing. Policy makers want physicians to be gatekeepers of society's resources and instruments of the bureaucratic apparatus; patients seek autonomy and see physicians increasingly as instruments of their wishes; ethicists question the value of the physician's fiduciary role—suggesting to some extent the adoption of a contractual arrangement between patient and physician; and administrators of managed care systems want physicians to be entrepreneurs, competitors, and instruments of profit.[1]

The capabilities of the physician are demeaned, on the one hand, as too technological, while at the same time physicians are unrealistically endowed by patients with magical powers that render them liable for the fallibilities of nature, which are often unforeseeable and sometimes unavoidable. To state the obvious, in treatment, things don't always go well, no matter the correctness of the plan or the skill with which it is implemented; yet the physician often shoulders the blame. Essentially, medicine is practiced in an atmosphere in which all that goes wrong must be blamed on someone. Fiscal incentives and disincentives are used as levers to modify physicians' behavior, and then the physician is chastised for responding. Finally, I hear with increasing frequency how patients have come to not feel any responsibility to the doctor, instead viewing the payment of the doctor as a matter between a third-party payer and the physician—the care being an entitlement.

Other forces are also at work in this kaleidoscope of interweaving demands that have been imposed on the practicing doctors. Underlying the turbulence of a fluid medical system is the obvious economic pressure created by the increasing cost of health care. A discussion of what is needed to fix these problems is not part of the mission of this book, but clearing up misconceptions by finding common understanding between the profession and the public certainly is. Thus, my need to point out that the steady rise of health care cost is to a large extent unrelated to a physician's fees. Doctors currently work as intensively as ever, but many do so for less money for the same effort. Considering the huge expense of a medical education, the long and arduous training required, and the many sacrifices and demands of the lifestyle, when coupled with the assumption of the extraordinary responsibility for human life, it is absurd for physicians not to be paid well. Before relegating the average doctor to a substantially lessened income, the public should contemplate the consequences. I will concede that, with some obvious exceptions, doctors do make a good living. Why shouldn't they? If a young person seeks wealth, however, I would not recommend the medical profession. To state the obvious, other careers are more financially attractive, and furthermore, attaining wealth should not be the reason for becoming a physician.

All of these influences must be dealt with by today's physicians, and all in a society with a compromised trust of authority figures, a tendency for social cynicism, and even moral pluralism. Why is it surprising to anyone that such an atmosphere potentially distracts from a doctor's primary mission, which is to render service and care for sick people? As a sequel to this line of thinking, it seems reasonable to ask whether moral integrity can ever be rescued from such an unpromising climate. Pellegrino believes the answer to this question is obvious. He contends that rescue it we must, and the healing relationship between physician and patient ought to serve as the moral fulcrum—the Archimedean point, if you will—from which the balance between self-interests and high medical standards must be struck.[2]

It is intuitive to me that in order to achieve this state, we must think of the profession as being in a higher realm—not in an elitist, but an idealistic way—than the rest of society. Accordingly, we must require a higher level of morality for its members. Some physicians resent being held to a different standard. Given what they believe to be the unwarranted and unfair infringements on the profession, they feel that survival behavior ought to be geared more to ground-level combative interaction. My contention, however, is that it diminishes the profession to respond negatively and allow our standards and especially our behavior to become average as we attempt to "work the system." Rescue of moral integrity can only lie in taking the high ground. So, answering the question that I posed in the first sentence of this chapter: yes, the public should hold physicians to a higher standard, and furthermore, we should be honored by that distinction.

How might the quest for such a standard translate into practical language? For starters, there should be specific actions that make the goals of our profession clear: Our leadership must somehow convince the public that the flawed system in which we labor is actually as much to the detriment of patients as it is to us. The inability of the profession to communicate this basic message has been a major failure on our part. It is fundamental that patients understand that we are in this together. The profession as a whole should stand for what is good, and follow a code that consistently recognizes that right is always right, and wrong is never right. The profession should admit complicity in some of what ails us—to some extent, in attempting to "work the system," we have forfeited the high ground and thus have brought some of our difficulties on ourselves. The profession should refute all attempts to devalue the lives of the vulnerable that happen to have mental, psychiatric, or physical compromise. The profession should promote care for all of the sick and wanting—should provide care for the uninsured—and should universally accept Medicare and Medicaid. Finally, and very importantly, all physicians and especially the leadership of the profession should consistently and unequivocally condemn our colleagues who function as moral pygmies by fraudulently exploiting the system, or by the ethical compromise of charging exorbitant fees and collecting them by manipulation of the coding systems to gain larger-than-warranted insurance payments.

The dishonor of physicians should be viewed with the same revulsion reserved for any betrayal of sacred trusts. For these individuals, the respectability automatically afforded by membership in the medical profession is but a transparent fig leaf covering unworthiness. Unless our stance on this is strong and steady, the ideals Pellegrino cites will not be realized. And although most of what I have said relates to medicine in general, because the thrust of this book concerns the psychic forces between cancer physicians and cancer patients, I will risk melodrama by adding that because cancer is associated with a unique patient vulnerability, an ethical breach while caring for this group of patients is especially despicable. In order to function effectively in this world of materialism and self-gratification, the physician must strike the proper balance—on the one hand, avoiding naiveté and behaving realistically, while also refusing to surrender those high ideals to which I have referred. The search for this balance has, to a large extent, been responsible for many of the vibrations in what ought to be a smoothly operating system. Despite the vibrations, however, I believe that moral standards are actually what will keep the system going, vibrations and all.

· 9 ·

A Practical Adaptation of the Original Oath in Search for Modern Relevance

$\mathcal{A}$t the dawn of history, the practice of medicine was based on magic and astrology, rather than on science. Hippocrates of Cos, who lived between the fourth and fifth centuries BC, was probably the first to insist upon both the scientific and the ethical aspects of medicine. It would, however, be inaccurate to think that the Hippocratic Oath as we know it generally represented Greek medical practice of the time. The Hippocratic thinking actually more resembled later Christian principles than the flexible Hellenistic practices of that time, in which infanticide, abortion, and suicide were condoned. It is thought, therefore, that Hippocrates essentially founded a new ethical way that earned him the title of *father of the profession*. Apparently, he proposed an oath that would be a nonbinding pledge of intent for ethical behavior in the practice of medicine. It has traditionally been recited collectively by graduating medical students during commencement exercises. I have a vivid memory of the excitement I felt when my first act after receiving the medical diploma was to recite the Oath with my classmates. The recitation of the Hippocratic Oath is, admittedly only a formality today, and it is done sporadically among institutions.

Many references are made to the Oath, but most patients and, surprisingly, some physicians have no idea what it actually says. I suspect that most people and many doctors think of it is as being of historic interest only—a writing that symbolizes a traditional rite of passage rather than a functional document. One of the essential messages of this book, however, is a negation of this idea and an assertion that much of this ancient but surprisingly precocious rule book is relevant and workable in today's practice of medicine— perhaps more so than in antiquity. Despite all of the various pressures of the times, there is an imperative for doctors to rescue the remnants of moral integrity from an unpromising climate. Because of my belief in the high ideals outlined in the Hippocratic Oath, and since this book deals with the issues of physician behavior and morality to a considerable degree, it is worth examining not only the Oath's original content, but also some of the modifications that have been made in a search for modern relevance.

Most medical schools administer some form of the Oath, usually tailored to bypass the original wording, which forbade abortion and euthanasia and essentially admonished physicians against performing surgery. It should be made clear, however, that the exclusion of statements on abortion and euthanasia from modern versions does not represent a de facto endorsement of either. The absence of the wording in reality allows legal flexibility, as well as debate and disagreement among members of the profession.

In fact, there is currently much vigorous dialogue within academic and legal circles on these matters. The issues of abortion and euthanasia in particular, and one other that relates to special surgical training, are actually within the dominion of this text, and with some exception, and without taking sides or endorsing a specific view, I will seek to weave the applicability of these topics into the reader's considerations. Obviously, other complex ethical issues that are associated with recently acquired knowledge are not in the original Oath—cloning and other genetic engineering, stem cell research, and others—all of which are appropriately of great interest to physicians and ethicists. However, a discussion that includes all necessary adaptations of the Oath is beyond the scope of this book which is primarily focused on cancer-related issues. Almost certainly, as scientific knowledge grows, new topics will arise that theoretically challenge the ethicists, and on a practical level challenge physicians who administer patient care. As this intellectual discourse evolves, the medical profession will almost certainly interact with, agree and disagree with, and oppose and acquiesce to the intellectual machinations of social anthropologists.

Because physician behavior is a recurrent theme throughout much of this book, we should examine Hippocrates's original document and spell out how it has been modified in search for modern applicability to contemporary physician behavior. In doing this, I have outlined only those changes that are relevant to cancer-related subjects. For example, certain adaptations, such as the Oath's restriction of abortion, is contentious today and warrants discussion, but for our purposes, only as it pertains to pregnancy in cancer patients, thus I have avoided a full discussion of that subject. Since guidance for a younger generation is fundamental to the mission of this book, my personal opinions are sometimes made obvious by way of anecdote, but they are not meant to challenge the reader's own beliefs. Hence, guidance in thoughtfulness rather than dictum is offered. To delve into the general discussion of abortion—thus venturing outside of the subject of cancer—would be presumptuous on my part and moreover would risk political polarization and dilution of the thoughts that are essential to my literary purpose.

The following is the full Hippocratic Oath that was originally translated from the Greek:

"I swear by Apollo, Asclepius, Hygeia, and Panacea, and I take to witness all the gods, all the goddesses to keep according to my ability and my judgment, the following Oath.

1. To consider dear to me, as my parents, him who taught me this art; to live in common with him and, if necessary, to share my goods with him; to look upon his children as my own brothers, to teach them this art.
2. I will prescribe regimens for the good of my patients according to my ability and my judgment and never do harm to anyone.
3. I will not give a lethal drug to anyone if I am asked, nor will I advise such a plan. Similarly I will not give a woman a pessary[1] to cause an abortion.
4. I will preserve the purity of my life and my art.
5. I will not cut for stone, even for patients in whom the disease is manifest; I will leave this operation to be performed by practitioners, specialist of this art.
6. In every house where I come I will enter only for the good of my patients, keeping myself far from all intentional ill-doing and all seduction, especially from the pleasures of love with women or men, be they free or slaves.
7. All that may come to my knowledge in the exercise of my profession or in daily commerce with men, which ought not to be spread abroad, I will keep secret and will never reveal.
8. If I keep this oath faithfully, may I enjoy my life and practice my art, respected by all men in all times; but if I swerve from it or violate it, may the reverse be my lot."

The first part of the original Hippocratic Oath that referred to the pagan gods is of course absent from modern day versions, as is the first paragraph that addresses "teaching medicine to the sons of my teachers." This section refers to the perpetuation of the guild of medicine in which the sons of physicians often followed in the family tradition. Until recent times, medical schools generally gave preferential consideration to the male children of physicians. The demography of medicine has, however, changed substantially—slowly in the 1970s, but dramatically in the last twenty to thirty years, so that now the selection process is largely based on a system of meritocracy, and as a result, at least half of the typical incoming classes are women. As the medical profession assumes more and more of a bi-gender personality, the cancer teams will undoubtedly also change. As with all parts of the "work force," the ramifications of this trend in terms of behavior provide fertile ground for discussion, which I happily leave to the social anthropologists and other scholars in behavioral biology. Thus, this part of the Oath no longer can be applied in the literal manner.

The section of the Oath that speaks of "never cutting for stone" (part 5) literally refers to the surgery that was done for kidney and bladder stones. This restriction was predicated on the fact that physicians of that time compromised their status in society if they did surgery, which was left to other less serious individuals. Surgical tasks were left largely to barbers. A contemporary interpellation and application, however, can be used for the restriction of surgery to those properly trained to do it. Taking this one step further in the discussion of cancer, one of the points made in this book is that in this day of very sophisticated cancer care, the multidisciplinary team of cancer specialists is the norm rather than the exception. As an integral part of that team, the surgical oncologist (i.e., the tumor surgeon) is key. Essentially, there is no place in cancer surgery for a surgeon with marginal training or one who does only occasional tumor surgery. In smaller communities, this issue creates much practical difficulty for both patients and local physicians, and when patients in smaller communities cannot or will not go to a cancer center, it can create a difficult dilemma for the local doctors.

Parts 2 and 3 of the Oath concern what is referred to in the modern parlance of bioethicists as "patient beneficence," or what might be loosely defined as that which is in a patient's best interest. "To prescribe regimens for the good of my patients . . . and never do harm to anyone" and "never give a lethal drug" are directives clear in their intent. This is the section of the Oath most relevant to the care of today's cancer patients, and as such to this book. Death and dying, physician-assisted dying, physician-assisted suicide, and euthanasia are important and often contentious issues that fall within this category. A substantive discussion of cancer care must involve these matters, and members of the cancer team should attempt to understand their own feelings regarding these sober issues. I compare this self-appraisal of the cancer doctor to the development of a psychiatrist, who is required to undergo personal therapy/analysis time as a patient with a psychiatric colleague. By undergoing this "analysis," they hopefully better understand how their own psychic strengths and limitations intersect those of their psychiatric patients. A comparable concept and dynamic are at work in oncology. Only after the physician has defined his or her own thoughts on death and dying should such a dialogue begin with a patient. Patients are often frightened of such a discussion and will not broach the subject. The possibility of death is at least a subliminal part of what lurks in the mind of most cancer patients, and when indicated, no one should be better able than an oncologist to delve into this. The avoidance of this uncomfortable discussion leads to misunderstandings, false assumptions and expectations, as well as a flawed approach to the patient's illness. Ideally, the effectiveness of the physician's communicative skills should mitigate the negativity of this most sober of topics.

Part 3 of the Oath prohibiting the induction of an abortion is deleted from the modern versions, not because the American medical profession endorses or condones the practice but in order to allow a discussion of this very contentious matter. In fact, the practice, while legal, is neither prohibited nor encouraged by the current guidelines of the profession. The subject deserves targeted discussion in this particular book, however, because obviously pregnancy and cancer are not mutually exclusive, and when a pregnant woman develops cancer, or when a cancer patient becomes pregnant, heart-wrenching decisions are sometimes required. In this circumstance, there is no place for an indecisive cancer doctor. In such an undesirable situation, it is not enough for the doctor to say, "Here are your options, but I don't have a recommendation—what you do, is up to you." Of course, it is "up to you," but in this situation a pregnant cancer patient is dominated by family and social influences, their own considerable fear of cancer, their preconditioning regarding the morality of abortion, and the hormonal instincts to protect the pregnancy that result from millions of years of evolution. For the cancer physician not to offer clear advice that might help a woman decide what to do is to shirk an important responsibility. Despite the fact that the "right" or the "wrong" of the matter depends on personal beliefs of the patient, it is incumbent on the cancer physician to lead the discussion, and in the process of doing that, lend their own opinion on the matter. The hardest question for the physician is "Doctor, what would you advise if this occurred in your family? Would you recommend that the pregnancy be terminated if I were your daughter?" In other words, the physician should weigh in on the discussion, and above all, be able to answer the very fair question that I have just theorized. It is important to distinguish what I might recommend and what one of my daughters would actually do. As intelligent and independent individuals, they would, of course, decide that on their own.

One of the important themes permeating the core of this book is the importance of patients' trust of their doctor and as a result of that trust, the enormous responsibility that is de facto bestowed on the physician. The physician must be careful to give advice that is totally unselfish and is in the best interest of the patient, that is to say, is based on beneficence. So while it is correct to be forthright in telling a patient what you would recommend for your own family, it is entirely inappropriate to exceed that in an attempt to convince the patient to breach his or her own moral code on something as important as the termination of a pregnancy. To paraphrase an old cliché: Be careful what you recommend to people, they may do it. And once it is done, you own part of the consequences.

No matter what the physician's bias, the discussion of both sides of the issue should be put forth as objectively as possible. If the choice of abortion is repugnant and unacceptable to the physician for personal reasons—religious or otherwise—that should be made clear, but in doing so, the physician must not create a judgmental atmosphere that thwarts the patient's decision-making ability. If that's not possible, another physician should be brought into the discussion. Conversely, if the physician recommends termination and is unable to support the patient's refusal to follow that advice, no matter how illogical it might seem to the physician, then new medical leadership should be sought. Throughout this book, the issue of patient autonomy appears and reappears, and this particular theoretical example exemplifies as well as any, the definition of this important contemporary concept.

Over many years of dealing with patients, I have come to realize that most cancer physicians don't begin to realize how powerful their influence really is. Frightened patients are especially vulnerable, and when a trusted physician pushes in one direction, real power is in play. This is especially problematic in a pregnant woman who has cancer. There are conflicts within such a patient that are almost unimaginable. In a way, the primordial instincts of maternal protectiveness are juxtaposed to the equally primordial instinct for survival, and when one adds the woman's sense of responsibility to her other children and her spouse, the dilemma can be paralytic. In this particular situation, parents and spouse are often unhelpful, since, understandably, their concern is more often than not skewed in favor of the mother. Thus, the trusted physician has extraordinary influence over a frightened patient, and it must never be exploited to promote values that are not beneficent. To do so is a form of betrayal.

I am haunted by the memory of a situation in which I may have been guilty of this very transgression. Early in my career, I cared for a patient with cancer who had first learned of a fairly large thyroid mass at the same visit to her obstetrician in which she was told that she was pregnant. Though the joy of hearing of the pregnancy was somewhat mitigated by the discovery of the mass, she and her husband were filled with anticipation of this, their first child. She was thirty-five years old and had been pregnant once before, but lost the baby in the first trimester. For five years following the miscarriage, she and her husband had tried in vain to conceive again; therefore, this pregnancy was a very welcomed event. The obstetrician referred her to me. Cytology analysis clearly showed a thyroid malignancy that contained aggressive features, but not to an extreme degree. I recommended a total thyroidectomy followed by radioactive iodine administration. Enter the consideration of the pregnancy.

This couple was prone to excitability and substantial anxiety, and they amplified each other's fears to a state of cancer terror. The obstetrician was somewhat passive in the process and basically turned the issue over to me. Given the absence of his input, the patient and her spouse eagerly anticipated my advice. This was a heady experience for a professionally immature young man, perhaps with a somewhat overblown sense of self-importance, and I unhesitatingly made a strong case for termination of the pregnancy prior to commencing the treatment strategy. After making it clear that they dreaded doing this, a sad and somewhat guilt-ridden couple relented to my dogmatic persistence and agreed to a therapeutic abortion. While not actually twisting arms, I now realize that I subverted patient autonomy by not objectively presenting all sides of the issue.

Several weeks later, I removed the patient's thyroid gland, and to my surprise, the pathology report showed a low-grade papillary carcinoma that by the standard of today or even then, could have been left alone until later in the pregnancy, when surgery would have been safe for the fetus. Furthermore, the radioactive iodine treatment could have either been avoided or, at a minimum, delayed until after the delivery. In my youthful exuberance to cure this woman, I had overreacted to a low-risk cancer, but more importantly, I had failed to think in-depth about all of the ramifications of my recommendation.

It is a cruel fact that this woman was never again able to conceive. I have made the point that when a treatment strategy is wrong, no matter how unfortunate the outcome, if the physician made a beneficent decision—that is to say, it was done with the genuine belief that it was best for the patient—it is more forgivable. Even today, what haunts me is not the possibility that perhaps I made an error in judgment—most doctors are guilty of that at some point—but the thought that my motives may not have been beneficent. Were vanity and dogmatism—both akin to arrogance—part of the algorithm that led to my recommendation? I hope not, although I suspect as much. I'll never know, nor will I forget.

Thankfully, the discovery of a cancer during pregnancy or the occurrence of a pregnancy in a patient being treated for cancer are both infrequent situations, but when it does happen, the oncologist's responsibilities differ from that of the obstetrician. With the latter, there are two primary patients. The cancer physician, on the other hand, has one main focus—mom is first and foremost, and in this author's opinion, should get the priority over the baby.

This view is strongly contrary to that of the teaching of the Roman Catholic Church, which clearly assigns equal value to the lives of the mother and baby. Essentially, Roman Catholic teaching is that all human life must be respected and protected absolutely from the moment of conception. Traditional Jewish theology, on the other hand, differs somewhat, not encouraging abortion, but considering the life and well-being of the mother to be the primary focus. As such, in situations in which cancer care of a pregnant patient is potentially compromised, an abortion is tolerable. Religious scholars of the various theologies have considered this matter extensively, but in the final analysis, it is the treating doctor and the patient who must make the intensely personal decision. Depending on the personalities involved, this is sometimes simple. More often, however, it provokes profound introspection, and during the course of all of this, it is important that the treating physician provide steady and strong leadership. As I mentioned earlier no matter how strongly the cancer physician's feelings on the relative value of the lives of mother and baby, there must be objectivity in outlining patient options. If the physician is not able to do this, a referral to another oncologist is in order.

A vigorous and often contentious debate continues within American society over the issue of whether an abortion is ever justified. Even though the United States Supreme Court has upheld a woman's right to choose in *Roe v. Wade*,[2] there remains a large segment of the population that feels otherwise. In fact, a Gallup poll done in May 2009 reported that 51 percent of Americans polled call themselves pro-life (antiabortion) rather than pro-choice (mother's choice) on the issue of abortion. An April 2009 Pew Research Center poll showed a softening of support for legalized abortion compared to the previous years of polling. People who said they support abortion in all or most cases dropped from 54 percent in 2008 to 46 percent in 2009. That the country is deeply divided over the legality of abortion is reflected by the fact that 23 percent of those polled in the Gallup study say it should never be legal and 22 percent say it should be legal under all circumstances.

On one extreme of the debate are certain groups such as the Roman Catholic Church that are unequivocally pro-life, and on the other end of the opinion spectrum, there are those who believe that abortion should be available on demand. Finally, some find a compromise position in which first-trimester abortion is permissible in certain select situations, such as in cases of rape or incest or if the mother's life is at high risk.

As it pertains to all abortion, therapeutic or otherwise, the Roman Catholic Church has always looked upon the life of the mother and the life of the unborn child as equal in value. Essentially, from the first moment of existence, a human being must be recognized as having the rights of a person.

The moment of conception, according to Catholic doctrine, is the completion of fertilization; when the zygote is formed, that is the new human organism.

Catholic doctrine includes what is known as the principle of double effect. This doctrine governs situations in which one action is followed by two effects, one good (and intended), the other foreseen but not intended. There are four specific conditions that govern this principle, and when those conditions are met, in certain situations—for example, treating a pregnant woman for uterine cancer—it is acceptable to perform the action even though it will lead to the death of the fetus (Latin for offspring). In other words, the principle of double effect justifies some good actions that also have bad consequences under certain conditions. Removing a cancerous uterus from a pregnant woman produces a tragic side effect in the termination of the pregnancy, but assuming there is no other less harmful option, the act is good, although the death of the fetus is not. The essence of this principle is that even if the loss of the child is expected, the action is acceptable if the primary intent was not to abort the baby but to treat the mother. This is a totally different from performing an abortion on a woman under cancer treatment who has become pregnant or a situation in which the already pregnant woman develops cancer, neither of which falls within the governance of the principle of double effect, but is strictly contrary to Roman Catholic doctrine. Simply put, intended abortion, no matter the circumstances, is never permitted within this doctrine.

Other criteria for the principle of double effect are equally important. I will discuss them briefly in another chapter; however, a full discussion of these very important tenets, which govern such a large number of both laypeople and the physicians caring for them, is well beyond the scope of this book. The reader is referred to a recently published book called *Catholic Health Care Ethics* for in-depth scholarship.[3] Cynics might contend that this principle of double effect is merely playing with words in order to enable Catholics to circumvent the essence of the issue. I leave this to the judgment of others.

Much of the public discussion (as opposed to legal) on abortion—whether the procedure is therapeutic or for convenience—centers on the question of whether or not a fetus is yet a person—thus the question of when life actually begins. The pro-choice advocates have concluded that an abortion does not really violate human life, and the pro-lifers contend that since life begins at conception, the violation is absolute. The Court's decision legalizing abortion did not dwell on the issue of the beginning of life, but instead focused on the "point of viability," which constituted that point beyond which the fetus would be able to sustain extrauterine life, with or without support. It is not my purpose to delve into the legal language of that ruling; that's for legal scholars and well beyond my reach and ability. Rather, I seek to point out that certain science is irrefutable: after fertilization (conception), there is continuous biologic growth, so by the time of implantation in the uterine wall at nine or ten days there is much going on within the fertilized egg, which by then is called an embryo. By the eighth week after conception a permanent genetic code exists, and the embryo is referred to as a fetus. The primitive skeleton and a functional cardiac system exist in this two-inch-long phenomenon, and, importantly, it responds to touch and is even capable of thumb sucking.

For me, when life actually starts is a nonissue. The question yields nothing more than repetition of what has been defined and redefined. To quote the Random House College Dictionary, life is "the general or universal condition of human existence." Referring to the product of conception as a fetus rather than a baby may constitute medically precise terminology, but when used to support a pro-abortion agenda, it is a scripted word alteration designed to depersonalize a human being. Whether considered right or wrong, justified or not, abortion should be labeled for what it really is—the taking of a human life. To think otherwise is to deny science. And in the wise words of Citizen John Adams (i.e., before he became president), "Facts are stubborn things; and whatever may be our wishes, our inclinations, or the dictates of our passions, they cannot alter the state of facts and evidence."

On the several occasions in which I have recommended a therapeutic first-trimester abortion in a cancer patient, I have thought of it as justifiably ending a life. That should not suggest that it was without a heavy emotional price for me, and truth be known, recommending an abortion always generated a real sense of remorse within me. After all, why should such a death be any less significant than that claimed in capital punishment or euthanasia? The point to be made is that while there are marked differences in the social implications of these three acts, there is also commonality among them. In point of fact, taking a life, whether in the uterus, the gas chamber, or a suite for administering a deadly potion during the act of euthanasia, should be labeled for what it really is—killing a human being on behalf of a person, a society, or an ideal. Justification for any or all of these is an entirely different topic for discussion. In the case of abortion, how one labels the product of conception doesn't make it any less alive or less human, nor does it make the act any less than killing. It is one of the major contradictions of contemporary times that there are intelligent people who are strongly pro-choice but who are appalled by the act of capital punishment. Until we can begin to look at human life as commencing with conception and ending with the cessation of biologic forces within, these issues will never be evaluated on a level playing field.

At the risk of sounding sinister, what is appropriately meant to protect secular governance in America has been clouded by an effort by some to desensitize the public to killing and to the assistance of killing, which is a process historically counterbalanced by ethics, laws, and the principles of the medical profession. Actually, the balance of social thinking was significantly altered by the 1973 ruling of the Supreme Court in *Roe v. Wade*, which legalized the killing of the unborn. Since then, many physicians and a portion of society have become increasingly desensitized to abortion in the early, middle, and even late stages of pregnancy. Abortion on demand is the norm now, rather than the exception. Partial birth abortion, in effect politically softer lingo for infanticide, is the extreme in stretching the limits of what was originally intended by the Court. In 2011 there was media sensationalism about the murder trial and conviction of a man who assassinated a doctor in Wichita, Kansas, who had been performing numerous late-term abortions. The media coverage brought to light that this procedure was performed more often than previously thought.

As part of medical training, doctors are conditioned to sights and occurrences that repel laypeople—autopsies, cadaver dissections, gruesome trauma, and so on—that type of conditioning goes with the territory and is unavoidable, even desirable. It is critical, however, that doctors not allow this state of desensitization to advance to the point of tolerance for that which is clearly wrong. As a means of lending realism to the possibility of insidiously crossing that line, one need look no further than the shameful complicity of physicians with Nazi sadism in the 1930s and 1940s when medical experimentation and murder were imposed on Gypsies, Jews, the disabled, the mentally challenged, and others. As it pertains to the discussion of abortion in the United States, even though the pro-choice faction prefers not to discuss this issue in the same context as euthanasia and capital punishment, in fact the outcomes are essentially the same. Attempting to justify any one of the three—abortion, euthanasia, or capital punishment—by minimizing the solemnity of the action is to wrap the issue in a type of intellectual delusion that diminishes the sanctity of life. The medical profession must neither passively nor actively encourage further erosion of the value that our society assigns to human life. In saying this, I am reminded of the words of the English author, John Donne (1572–1631) that were put in a modern form by Ernest Hemingway, "Any man's death diminishes me, because I am involved in Mankind; and therefore never send to know for whom the bell tolls; it tolls for thee."[4]

When a pregnant woman develops cancer, or when a cancer patient who is under treatment becomes pregnant, those that advocate therapeutic abortion justify it because of their concern that the cancer treatment places the unborn child at risk of serious birth defects or mental damage or that optimal treatment of the mother is compromised by the pregnancy. This posture is abhorrent to many, however, and Roman Catholic doctrine unequivocally refutes it. Even though the issues of birth defects and fetal injuries from nuclear energy and anesthetic and chemotherapeutic agents are far more than theoretical, and are real possibilities with which the physician and the family must deal, the orthodox pro-life way of thinking contends that possible or even probable injury to a fetus does not legitimize its eradication. To protect victims from potential harm by killing them is counterintuitive. The very basic question in this line of thinking: Is there harm worse than death?

With this overview of the pertinent facts, I will analyze practical details regarding termination of a pregnancy that is motivated by the development of maternal cancer. In doing research for this book, I had discussions with other oncologists—surgical, radiation, and medical—whose collective expertise covered most malignancies. In my particular career, I have dealt almost exclusively with cancers of the head and neck, and because many of these malignancies occur in older people, the coexistence of pregnancy in this subset of patients is unusual. There are, however, malignancies that occur in the head and neck area that are neither age nor gender specific. They require various types of therapy, some of which can cause fetal damage. Cancer of the thyroid and salivary glands, nasopharynx, and tonsils; malignant melanoma; sarcomas; and lymphopoietic malignancies often require various combinations of surgery, systemically administered nuclear radiation, external beam radiation, or chemotherapy.

After considering all of the above—head and neck as well as the malignancies of other areas—I am struck by how seldom abortion is even a consideration, even by those unopposed to the practice. Essentially, what would seem to be an often-encountered problem is, in fact, an unusual occurrence. When it occurs, however, the dilemma must be faced with a well-thought-out philosophy. First of all, even in situations in which the fetus will be directly exposed to drugs and/or nuclear energy, the requirement is never absolute. In other words, a mother can and frequently does reject the notion of abortion, either because of religious conviction or simply in response to protective maternal instincts. More frequently, however, the cancer team is able to circumvent the problem by delaying the use of chemotherapy or nuclear energy until later in the pregnancy when the developmental impact on the fetus is minimal. In less aggressive cancers such as most thyroid lesions, surgery can be delayed until the middle trimester, and then, if radioactive iodine is required, it can be administered after the baby is born. Breast cancer is probably the most common malignancy that occurs during pregnancy, and its management can usually wait for at least moderate fetal development.

In those cancers that appear to be highly aggressive—acute leukemia, some lymphomas, some breast cancers, or others in which early employment of aggressive therapy is essential—the difficult decision of whether to terminate the pregnancy presents itself. The precision of modern radiation therapy planning has made the delivery of external beam radiation with protection of the fetus more feasible. There are still circumstances, however, in which the scatter effects of abdominal and thoracic radiation theoretically have a detrimental effect on fetal development and perhaps on development of cancers later in the life of the child. For me, there is no generic right or wrong. It is rather the responsibility of all concerned to understand the potential impact on the unborn and to follow one's conscience in the decision process. I believe that the wishes of the parents, and especially the mother, are paramount—and the physician's lead in education and recommendations is critical to an informed decision.

The standards for what is harmful to a first-trimester fetus fluctuate. Over the years, a number of drugs thought harmless in this setting—for example, thalidomide, tetracycline, and certain vitamins—have ultimately been responsible for birth defects. Even some over-the-counter drugs that were previously thought harmless to early pregnancy have been found to have hurtful consequences to fetal development. So I am skeptical of the reassurance that chemotherapy during pregnancy can be safely delivered. Certainly, the timing of drug delivery can minimize fetal damage, but even ideal timing fails to eliminate my skepticism.

Up to this point, I have expounded mostly from an objective point of view—pointing out facts and quoting from medical and religious doctrine. At this juncture, however, I ask the reader's indulgence of a subjective discussion of the psycho-metabolic forces that I believe are at play in both mother and child during pregnancy. The consideration of these important factors has instinctively influenced my feelings on the coexistence of pregnancy and maternal cancer, and I put my thinking forward for the reader to mull over. During the amazing biologic event of pregnancy, there are extraordinary hormonal and protective influences that occur within the mother, and the bonding that develops between mother and the intrauterine child, while not measurable, is admittedly profound. Certain facets of evolutionary biology that have developed over millions of years are at full throttle during these developmental months. Even though other people are able to peripherally share in this phenomenon, the experience is singular and extraordinary for a woman. In point of fact, pregnancy is the quintessential female experience. With that said, I'm fully aware that the extreme of the stress on a woman's body during the full term is truly remarkable.

Although I cannot substantiate it scientifically, it is intuitive to me that maternal psychic and metabolic forces—both of which are related to the autonomic nervous system—are inextricably interactive with those of the fetus. I believe that many of the mother's chemicals—those associated with her anxieties, her fears, and her mood cycles—are transmitted to the baby. My suspicion is that the fetus is able to perceive at some level that the pregnancy is happy and welcomed or, conversely, unwanted and dreaded. Obviously, there are some chemicals that do not cross the placental barrier, and this statement admittedly is a huge generalization, but fundamentally, the obvious question is, how does all of this influence our discussion of cancer management?

My answer is that ideally the mother's psychic and metabolic energy should be concentrated on the task of pregnancy, and that a cancer constitutes an enormous distraction and metabolic competition—at a minimum, emotional turmoil. It follows, then, that when this coincidence in timing occurs, neither the pregnancy nor the fight against the cancer can receive the full complement of targeted energy. Within that same line of thought, I approach cancer like a war, and the battles involve a total marshalling of the body's defenses. I want a patient to focus on fighting the war, and it seems to me that a pregnancy dilutes the intensity of that mission.

In the planning stages of cancer treatment of nonpregnant women who are of childbearing age, I always counsel the patient to avoid pregnancy during the treatment time and for at least one year after its completion. The whole "cancer experience" is so emotionally and physically demanding that even with successful treatment an extended recovery time is required to begin to feel well again. I have a very blunt and specific discussion with the partner of such a patient, and with both man and woman present, place the responsibility for strict birth control on both of them. Personal involvement and leadership by the cancer physician are important at this juncture, and I make a point to challenge the man to strictly adhere to his part of the covenant. Depending on my interpretation of the couple's relationship and on their level of maturity, I might even say to the male, "She has enough to worry about without being concerned with getting pregnant. I'm counting on you to make sure this does not happen—OK?" The OK question is not asked casually. With direct eye contact between the man and me, I wait for his acquiescence, either with a positive nod or verbal compliance. This commitment to absolute birth control—abstinence if necessary—is especially important during the treatment, but it is not as simple as it sounds. Certain orthodox segments of both the Jewish and the Roman Catholic populations are vigorous in their opposition to any interference with the normal reproductive cycle. In observant women, the consultation of a rabbi or a priest is recommended, and a game plan suitable to all concerned is developed. Sexual urges nevertheless sometimes win out over a pledge to rationality, and mistakes are made; hence, unplanned pregnancies happen. These are particularly problematic during the treatment period, and one must revert to the abortion discussion. The unplanned pregnancy that occurs after treatment but during the first year that I had assigned for observation is less of a problem. Generally, a positive attitude, a congratulatory gesture, and "moving on" are all that is employed. Scorn or reprimand at this juncture are not useful; better to keep a positive and affectionate relationship rather than risk ill will.

In all situations, the mother's feelings regarding this whole matter are paramount. Below I describe three real-life examples of patients that I cared for, all of whom had different situations—different cancers, different life circumstances, and different attitudes about abortion.

Example 1: During the 1970s, I saw a young woman who had a mass that was deeply imbedded in her neck, lying under her mandible. The X-rays were suggestive of an aggressive malignancy, although she only had minimal symptoms. This twenty-five-year-old woman was accompanied by her husband of two years. She had just missed a menstrual period, and a subsequent test revealed an early pregnancy. This was her first pregnancy and because this couple wanted a family, given different circumstances, this would have been a welcomed event. They were in agreement, however, with the notion that the mother's welfare was to be the first priority in this situation. The combination of surgical excision, postoperative radiation, and chemotherapy was to be the treatment strategy of choice, and the ominous appearance of the tumor made time of the essence.

Obstetricians and anesthesiologist agree that to do general anesthesia and operate at a very early stage of pregnancy is somewhat unsafe for the fetus, and when we do have to operate on a pregnant woman, we reluctantly do so only in the middle trimester, thus allowing important early development of the baby to be unencumbered. In this particular patient, waiting for two and a half months would have been unwise. The patient, the husband, the obstetric and also the pediatric consultants, and the patient's rabbi were all brought into the discussion, which was intelligent but understandably emotional. The recommendation to abort the baby prior to tumor surgery was unanimous among nonfamily. The mother and father made a sad but prompt decision. The pregnancy was terminated within two days, and the following week, major tumor surgery was done. The treatment strategy thought to be in the best interest of the mother was selected. Despite the full implementation of the strategy, however, the patient died of disseminated malignant disease the following year.

As I mentioned previously, Jewish doctrine generally considers the mother's condition to be paramount, and while not being casual about this very serious decision, most rabbis advise accordingly. Such is not the case with the Roman Catholic Church, in which the rights of both the mother and the unborn child are both sacrosanct and both must be protected to the extent possible. If the above example had occurred in an observant Catholic, most priests would have advised against the abortion, choosing instead to accept the risk to the child of early surgery or to the mother if she chose to wait until the middle trimester. If early surgery was done, and if the pregnancy was lost because of the surgery, that is, a miscarriage, that would have been unavoidable and sad but acceptable. I refer the reader back to my superficial discussion of the Roman Catholic doctrine known as the principle of double effect. Any treatment that would have placed the baby in harm's way would have been accepted as part of the risk. Obviously, if the opportunity to wait for fetal development before starting such treatment is an option, so much the better; however, such a course is fraught with risks in higher-grade or ominous tumors. Obviously, in low-risk tumors, there is less urgency in starting treatment. Even in the lower-grade malignancies, however, either with or without the advice of the cancer physician, the parents may opt for an abortion, preferring to intensely focus on the cancer combat that might be ahead. Such was the case in the next example.

Example 2: About ten years ago, I saw as a patient a forty-year-old woman who had been diagnosed with thyroid cancer and who happened to be in the early stages of her first pregnancy. She and her husband, a fellow physician, had married one year before, and because of her age, and her diminishing window of opportunity for pregnancy, they were delighted to know she was pregnant. The thyroid mass was discovered by her obstetrician at the time of the initial visit for the suspected pregnancy. The malignancy obviously muted the joy of the pregnancy. When I saw her, I found that she had a low-risk tumor—moderate in size and of the type that could have waited until the middle trimester of the pregnancy, at which time an operation that would have been safe for the baby would have probably cured the mother. I gave her the option of waiting for a mid-trimester operation or an immediate operation following a therapeutic abortion. I did not give her the choice of an immediate cancer operation.

The woman and her husband both wanted my advice, asking, "What would you recommend if I were your family?" I answered that because of the low-grade nature of the cancer there was no right or wrong approach but my best advice was to go ahead with the abortion and an early operation. I did not promote my advice but only answered the question as asked. My reasons for recommending this course of action were not related to the aggressiveness of the cancer; instead, as I have discussed in one of the preceding paragraphs of this section, I believe that "the cancer experience" is emotionally all-consuming and the time for focusing on treatment and the long period (one year or so) of uncertainty and emotional recovery is better served without the distraction of a pregnancy. In the process, neither the cancer nor the pregnancy gets the full intensity of effort. That was my opinion, and when asked, I offered it, although I was prepared to proceed with an alternative plan in which no abortion was done. As I said earlier, the doctor ought to be able to make a personal recommendation, regardless of the actual objective indications. There were no religious issues, and the patient and her husband decided to terminate the pregnancy.

The obvious implications of this woman's age were important, but did not outweigh the desire to have an uncomplicated period during which the cancer could be combated. Happily, after a successful operation and nuclear medical treatment, she went on to have a second pregnancy that introduced a healthy baby into an almost recovered family.

Example 3: This example involves a twenty-three-year-old woman who had a salivary gland cancer that was ominous looking and should have been treated aggressively and promptly. The patient was in an early stage of her first pregnancy and because of a strongly held belief that abortion was wrong absolutely would not even discuss the need to terminate the pregnancy and start vigorous treatment in a timely manner. Despite the general sense of urgency, her strong sense of responsibility for her baby precluded any other consideration. The husband was concerned for his wife, and he and I strongly urged her otherwise. Maternal protective instincts dominated, and I was clearly given a mandate from this young woman. "Doctor, I'll wait until it's safe for the baby to start treatment—period." End of discussion.

I removed the tumor about eight weeks later. The surgery was uneventful, and mother and fetus did well. Immediately following the term delivery of a healthy baby, postoperative radiation therapy was begun; thus the compromise imposed by the delays in both surgery and radiation therapy were recognized and accepted. Apparently, the delays were not critical, and she has stayed in touch with me for fifteen years, each year happily reporting that she and her son were doing very well. Obviously, relationships can be strained by such a dividing trauma, and in this case, she heard and ultimately rejected my strong advice regarding the pregnancy, following which, our doctor-patient relationship continued. Such was not the case with the young husband, who had failed to provide her with what she thought was real support. The marriage did not last. I am quick to point out that in this case, this brave young mother was right (and lucky), and I was wrong! I don't believe that she ever even considered my recommendations. The moral of the story is that the mother's wishes—not those of the doctor and not even those of her husband—should prevail.

· *10* ·

Death and Dying:
Natural and Otherwise

*Think not disdainfully of death, but look on it with favor; for even
death is one of the things that Nature wills.*

—*Marcus Aurelius*

*A*ny book that discusses the psycho-science of cancer must deal with death
and dying. This is especially so because cancer is no longer an automatic
death sentence. In fact, there are certain cancers, such as prostate, kidney,
bladder, thyroid, salivary gland, and others, in which certain subtypes of the
respective diseases can linger for years—even decades, in a metastasized state,
all the while making their presence known only as shadows on radiographic
images or scans. Because of these admittedly infrequent circumstances, cancer
jargon should be adapted to include the phrase *living with cancer*. Essentially,
such malignancies take on the imprimatur of a chronic disease, and not infrequently the patient goes on with a very functional lifestyle, ultimately dying
from another cause. Therefore, in this era in which we have the capability of
creating remission without cure, we must continually rethink the issues that
pertain to quality of life after treatment; and when the impotence of tumor
dormancy ends and tumor progression begins, the issues of quality of death
must take center stage in our thinking.

As this important distinction is considered, the relevant societal attitudes and laws that govern our ability to mitigate a patient's final exit
become very important. The ancient Oath by which physicians have lived
was developed when the biologic understanding of cancer was limited to
the comparison of its behavior to that of a crab (as in the Greek, Karkinos).
Therefore, historically prevalent thinking should be adapted to include
the contemporary attitudes toward life with cancer and life while dying.
I was tempted to include the forthcoming discussion in the chapter on

Adaptation of the Oath for Modern Relevance, just as I did with the subject of the coexistence of pregnancy and cancer. But because the subject is so much more extensive and consistently problematic, I have chosen to discuss death and dying separately and have included in this discussion difficult and contentious ethical topics. However, to jump into the essence of these subjects without linking them to historical precedent would be like discussing space travel without first talking about physics and astronomy. It is my belief that the cancer physician must demonstrate leadership in this arena, and as such, the various considerations explored in this chapter are important for the basis of individual philosophies. However, while the physician may provide guidance, the ultimate arbiter of a patient's issues of death and dying must be the patient. With this in mind, I hope that both the physician and the patient will benefit from the following discussion and that the mutual understanding they might gain can help circumvent misunderstanding and interpersonal difficulties.

The general topics of death and dying are profoundly complicated, and the endless debates that occur among scholars—philosophers, ethicists, sociologists, lawyers, and physicians—are often contentious, usually passionate, mostly opinionated and polarized, but rarely conclusive. Such issues as assisted dying, patients' right to a type of death of their choosing, doctors' responsibilities to their patients and to society regarding death and dying, patients' right to feel entitled to assistance in promoting their own death, and many other burning questions are pervasive in our changing system of values. The fact that there is often ambivalence and confusion among the public about the relevant moral issues therefore comes as no surprise; after all, it would be unrealistic to expect a society to comprehend easily what so many learned individuals have struggled to make sense of.

A cursory look at this complicated search for conclusions is revealing. Two different presidential commissions, a committee of the Harvard Medical School, the United States Supreme Court, various state courts, state legislatures, and many other bodies have struggled for years to reach consensus on various end-of-life issues, whether in cancer patients or otherwise. Consider the vast menu for study—euthanasia, physician-assisted death, the persistent vegetative state, brain death, and the applicability of the law in family disputes that involve not only these individual issues but also the implied role of medical technology. These and other personal and legal questions create a bewildering array of elusive considerations in a fluid social environment and value system that are both increasingly characterized by secularization, analytical thinking, and dependence on technology.

Although the overall thrust of this book focuses on cancer-related issues, these topics should concern all doctors, and it is vital that both individual physicians and the leadership of the profession provide guidance and direction in these great social debates. Throughout history, societal leaders have made important decisions and proclamations based only on the input of theorists rather than the participation of people who actually have to live with the rulings. Such has been the case with many of the radical changes that have occurred throughout the health care system, some of which have been beneficial and others extraordinarily ill advised and counterproductive.

The individual doctor is appropriately preoccupied with patient care, and because the leadership of the profession has not consistently been strong and dynamic, medical professionals have not always participated adequately in the discussions that lead to policy decisions. Because of this and other reasons, large corporations and the federal government have effectively taken control of the health care system. While this may be unpleasant for physicians, it is somewhat understandable, given the fact that we are not always wise in business or policy matters. This said, it's hard to imagine a messier design for a system than that in which we currently labor. Neither doctors nor patients are happy with it.

Lest we repeat the error of our ways, physicians must realize that control of many nonadministrative issues such as death and dying must be within the dominion of the profession. Since a rendezvous with death is common to all of humankind, shouldn't medical caregivers—the overseers of dying, as well as the final exit—be part of those discussions that standardize, regulate, and establish the ethics and the legal language applied to the process? I believe that we will be excluded from these social and legal debates if we avoid the hard work and intellectual tenacity that philosophers, ethicists, sociologists, and legal scholars bring to the discussion table. It is paradoxical that poets, legal scholars, theologians, and philosophers have written extensively about death and dying while the people who frequently witness death—doctors, nurses, hospice personnel, and others—rarely write about it.[1]

Whatever the extent of our participation in these discussions, it must be based on a practical brand of scholarship that possesses the underpinning of morality, humaneness, and an intense value for life. The legal profession has appropriately shared in the debate and, I might add, the confusion. For example, the U.S. Supreme Court's 1997 decisions in *Washington v. Glucksberg* and *Vacco v. Quill* held that there is no constitutional right to physician-assisted suicide, whether by passive participation or by direct infliction of death, but, in not ruling either for or against in the cases, the Court sidestepped the moral issue and left the path of resolution to the individual states.[2] Additionally, by this "nonruling," the court has encouraged the contentious and age-old question to surface—should there be one, and only one, law of the land? Or is an array of state laws okay?

Political forces have led to state referenda and sometimes to laws, such as in Washington State, Oregon, and Montana, in which the right to passively assist in suicide has been bestowed upon doctors. These referenda were held as a result of the U.S. Supreme Court's abdication, and as these particular state laws now stand, a doctor can assist in a patient's suicide in an advisory and preparatory capacity, that is, they can prescribe medication. However, in each case, the doctor is prohibited from actually attending the act. These laws stipulate that death must be requested by the patient, and importantly, they do not sanction active physician termination of life, such as in Holland, where a doctor can actually administer a lethal drug. In reality, the Dutch physicians are walking a fine line, because even there, while tolerated, the practice is technically illegal. When a physician-assisted death is reported, if strict guidelines are followed, the court "looks the other way." The United States law concerning the difference between physician-assisted suicide and active euthanasia is clear, however. This fact was vividly demonstrated by the travails of Jack Kevorkian, an anesthesiologist who participated in over a hundred physician-assisted suicides without major legal consequences. However, he was convicted of second-degree murder when he crossed the legal line by actively terminating the life of a patient, and then he dramatized and flaunted his disdain for the law by speaking of it on television. Kevorkian served eight years in prison.

Without trying to analyze what motivated Kevorkian, it is safe to say that his defiance not only put him at odds with the law but also with the stated policy of virtually every leadership organization in medicine. With the exceptions of Holland, Luxembourg, Belgium, and Colombia, the medical leadership of the developed countries in Europe, Asia, and the Americas has condemned the active participation of physicians in causing the death of a patient, no matter what may seem to be the justification, including a direct request by the patient to do so. This consensus alone should be enough for any physician to care for patients from birth to death unencumbered by ambivalence relative to this question. In this book, however, I have tried to deal with more than what is practical and also include right and wrong, moral obligations, empathy, personal emotions, understanding the psychic forces affecting cancer patients, and many others matters that flow through the core of this discussion. So it seems appropriate to discuss the huge topic of euthanasia, or mercy killing, in at least a condensed manner. Regardless of my personal feelings on this matter, to fail to stimulate a dialogue among the readership would be shirking my responsibility as an educator.

It is uncertain if legalization of active euthanasia will ever be proposed for public referendum, but what I do believe to be predictable is that such legalization will not occur without the contribution—through action or inaction—of the medical profession. This belief is predicated on what I mentioned earlier in discussing the importance of the profession's participation and leadership in such important social debates. If we fail to participate, we in effect risk complicity and even encouragement of whatever happens.

The word *euthanasia* is somewhat misunderstood. Contemporary usage equates it with the common term *mercy killing*. Actually, the word derives from the Greek *eu* ("easy") and *thanatos* ("death"). The ancient Greeks didn't specifically refer to active killing but applied it more generally, with the connotation of a good death—which to them was a death without pain. For the sake of clarity in these legally precise times, however, some standardization of nomenclature should be used, and during this discussion, I will refer to euthanasia as only the acceleration of the natural process of dying.

In contemporary jargon and literature, *active euthanasia* results from actions meant to directly cause death, as with the delivery of a lethal solution. *Passive euthanasia*, on the other hand, represents the allowance of death by withholding or withdrawing treatment. Technically speaking, suicide, whether assisted or unassisted, could be considered a form of self-imposed euthanasia. To avoid categorical complexity, however, it should be thought of and dealt with separately. Assisted suicide includes passive and active assistance. In the passive version, another person assists in the setup but is not present for the act, and obviously is not allowed to administer whatever is chosen for the instrument of death. In this setting, the person destined to die actually administers the potion. This is the version of assisted suicide permitted in the three northwestern states in America in which a doctor is able to write the prescription for the planned suicide that is to be accomplished by the patient. In active assisted suicide, another person, sometimes a doctor, sometimes not, administers the potion. In parts of Europe, such as in Germany and Switzerland, the active assistance of a person other than a doctor is accepted.

In those circumstances in which a physician is asked to participate in a patient's suicide, whether by assistance or only as passive spectator, and also in any situation in which a voter might be asked to judge a proposed change in the status of physician's involvement in death—such as happened in Oregon, Washington State, and Montana—the individual physician or layperson must not lose touch with what "feels" right and what "feels" wrong; those instincts are profound in people of substance and integrity, and they should be heeded. From my own personal standpoint, if an act or action feels wrong, then it usually turns out to be just that; that is to say, one's instincts tend to serve as an accurate moral compass. It has been said that wrong is always wrong, even when everyone is doing it; and right is always right, even if no one is doing it. While these statements may be overly simplistic given the complexity of contemporary social and human behavior, the spirit of the statements can be borrowed and employed.

Despite the shifting sands in the ongoing secularization of American society, physicians especially must tap into their instincts of right and wrong. Even though the public is often disappointed with the medical profession, the majority still want to idealize medical doctors and expect them to follow that which is right. Is it not intuitive that the public should be able to look to certain figures in which to find standards of integrity—and where better to look than the medical profession? After all, a physician's behavior should be founded on a simple and unselfish premise—service to humankind. And woe to the transgressors of this trust. Public disdain can be passionate for doctors who don't live up to a high standard, because when that happens, feelings of betrayal are created.

To cite the permanence of certain social stains, the civilized world remembers relatively recent German history in which a sophisticated, educated, and seemingly humane society began to devalue life, fertilized xenophobic hatred for religious and racial differences, discriminated against and devalued the handicapped, ridiculed and disrespected the mentally ill and retarded, and, ultimately, complied with and tolerated unthinkable acts of barbarism during the height of Nazi rule. Lest we as doctors skirt the real history, the German medical profession—not all, of course, but a significant part of it—was involved in some of the most hideous planning and behavior; and importantly, the silent inaction of the general physician population was itself tantamount to complicity.

This point cannot be made any clearer than Michael Burleigh's account in his sobering book about euthanasia in Germany in the first half of the twentieth century, *Death and Deliverance*.[3] The author writes of a gradual hardening of a particular moral climate and the slow depletion of a post-Christian and illiberal ideology. In this important work of eye-opening revelations, the basic question is asked as to why so many ordinary Germans abandoned concern for the weak in favor of a vulgar ideology of social Darwinism that dragged the whole society down to the laws of the jungle. Years later, despite Germans' searching for moral absolution through xenogenesis, financial reparation, admission of and contrition for crimes against humanity, the stain of guilt continues to permeate the core of that society. Importantly, because of the medical profession's complicity in euthanasia performed for reasons related to chronic medical and psychiatric illness, birth defects, retardation, and for human experiments, neither a place of honor within society nor the general trust of doctors has been completely restored in Germany. While the international community seems to have forgiven the German people, the medical profession's betrayal of the Oath was apparently judged by both the German people and the international community as a less forgivable descent into amorality. This seems appropriate to those of us who believe that physicians ought to be held to a higher moral and ethical standard than laypeople.

Burleigh's question of why so many ordinary people participated in and tolerated the inhumane acts being discussed was probably intended to apply to both physicians and laypeople; however, my suspicion is that the question is not entirely answerable. Nevertheless, there is an important practical point to be made: Just because these questions are beyond our comprehension doesn't mean that similar bad behavior won't reoccur. Nazism was like a mythological monster that inhaled its neighbors. Not content with the acquisition of *Lebensraum* ("living space"), the monster sadistically and systematically inflicted indignity and pain on countless human beings, and, important to my message, the medical profession was a willing part of the team. It is essential that each generation of doctors be taught this component of German history, otherwise, naive and unrealistic idealists will "govern us back" into complacency and a state of vulnerability.

It is especially important that knowledge of this particular history be at the foundation of the debate over euthanasia and physician-assisted suicide. Failing to learn from unpleasant history is a human tendency that has been with us since antiquity. Euripides (c. 485–406 BC) said, "Whoso neglects learning in his youth loses the past and is dead for the future."[4] I was reminded of this recently while reading a fascinating book by Bascomb, *Hunting Eichmann*,[5] that described a mind-set in Israel—even in the 1950s—in which public interest in finding and punishing war criminals was dramatically waning, and in an attempt to counter this, a concerted effort by less forgiving Israelis was required to resurrect memories of the Holocaust. Even among Israeli citizens, many of whom were concentration camp survivors, there was a tendency to move on and forget. While this analogy may seem a bit far-fetched, I believe it is relevant to the issues under discussion in this book because it demonstrates a consistent and dangerous human trait, which could be repeated as modern-day scholars consider the legalization of programmed killing of other humans, and while doing that, overlook just how cruel and hateful people can be.

I should confess that prior to doing research for this book, I suspected that the extent of physician complicity with the German euthanasia programs had been exaggerated. As it turned out, however, far from being hyperbole, the general story and the specific sins of the profession exceeded those I had known. Furthermore, I had been unaware of an attitude during the Weimar Republic that was similar to what existed during Nazi governance. The two periods are in fact connected by a not-so-subtle bridge of public tolerance and

support that culminated with the vulgarity and immorality of Nazis psycho-
pathology. The earlier period had set the stage for that which was magnified
just prior to World War II. An official program was sanctioned in 1939 by
the decree of Chancellor Hitler himself, in which patients—not prisoners,
mind you, but patients—were to be singled out because of certain chronic illnesses such as advanced cancers, tuberculosis, birth defects, severe disabilities,
insanity, retardation, epilepsy, schizophrenia, "perversions," and so on, and
were sent to various hospital-like facilities around Germany where they were
systematically murdered and cremated. The deceptions that were used for
the admission process were compounded by the creation of fraudulent death
certificates, and amazingly, the charade was topped off by fabricated letters
of condolence that were sent to the victim families in which their deaths were
blamed on an accident or a disease.

Although the program was carried out under the auspices of the National Socialist government, it would be inaccurate to think of it purely as a
Nazi endeavor; it was much more. Many of the involved physicians were not
even members of the Nazi party. Their deviation from the Oath to which
they were sworn led to a perversion of civilized behavior that fostered a credo
of eugenics and social engineering with a flair for the sadistic. The program
itself was conceived by lawyers and physicians, but importantly, was operated
by the latter. Incredibly, physicians actually carried out the killings! So that
the reader not dismiss these medical men as a rogue faction of psychopathic
misanthropes run amok, it should be pointed out that the program's spon-
sors and senior participants were leading medical professors and psychiatrists
in Germany, who were men of international reputation.[6] Euthanasia had
been discussed and debated in German society for sometime, and was no
more than a logical application of the principles of social Darwinism and the
budding science of eugenics. Physicians in this program alone killed almost
300,000 German citizens between 1939 and 1945. Importantly, these were
not Jews and Gypsies whose condemnation was predicated on other criteria,
but were citizens in good standing, who were not even necessarily terminally
ill or in unusual distress. Essentially, they were patients whose physicians had
decided their "lives not worth living"—which is a phrase officially created by
the generation that immediately preceded Hitler.

The pre-Nazi mind-set to which I refer partially ripened in the first
third of the twentieth century, and was driven to maturation by the economic
destitution that followed World War I. This was a time during which some
sociologists and leaders in government, law, and medicine looked to relieve
the bottom line by unburdening the economy of certain human ballast. After
a long period of expansion of Germany's commitment to asylums for the
retarded, the insane, and others in the first twenty years of the century, there

then came a major retraction of the nation's concern for the vulnerable. As early as 1920, economic imperatives were being articulated that addressed the inability of an impoverished state to support the type of mental asylum provisions that had previously existed in Germany. These words and others blended in with the crescendo of social dialogue related to the pseudo-science of eugenics and what I call euthanasia of convenience, as opposed to euthanasia based on idealism.

Most influential in the euthanasia debate of that time was the publication in 1920 of the work of Karl Binding, a leading German expert on constitutional and criminal jurisprudence and a noted academic.[7] In Binding's treatise, *Permission for the Destruction of Life Unworthy of Life*, he argued that the subject of involuntary euthanasia was no longer merely one of academic interest but that hard choices would have to be made about the allocation of scarce resources. At an important medical convention in 1921, a vigorous discussion took place on what to do with "life unworthy of life," and there was even a motion made before the general membership for the approval of euthanasia of patients whose lives were deemed "unworthy of life."[8] In Dresden the following year (1922), the program of the annual meeting of the Society of Forensic Psychiatry devoted an entire session to euthanasia of those "unworthy of life," and during the lengthy debate, one of the lead discussants argued that the money spent on "idiots" could be better used to prevent tuberculosis. His argument was extended to say, in effect, that pity was misplaced to include those in whom there was no subjective suffering.[9] Refutations invoked the Hippocratic Oath, which was then considered the gold standard for physician behavior. Even though the motion that was before the group was ultimately defeated, it is significant that an entire session of vigorous and earnest debate was expended on what turned out to be a harbinger of things to come with the next generation. Importantly, those promoting this eugenic prophylaxis were shameless in revealing their vision of the future. Notable Germans of the period other than physicians and legal scholars also publicly advocated this "societal modernization." For instance, a popular author of the time, Hoffmann,[10] used fiction to outline his vision of a eugenic dystopia in which he described roving commissions of doctors, armed with police powers and unencumbered by denunciation, who would select the unfit for elimination.

Almost certainly, there were ethical German physicians who were repelled by this relentless reversal of what medicine should stand for, but in the final analysis there does not seem to have been a unified stentorian objection from the medical community.

I would urge those readers who have a particular interest in this section to study two important and well-researched books—one by Gallagher and the other by Burleigh, both of which have been referenced considerably in this section. These books are shocking but well documented depictions of this evil and demented episode in German history.

Because there is already an extensive literature on euthanasia and related topics, it would be presumptuous for me to attempt more than an overview of this subject. Also, it's important to point out that the relevant debates and laws are so dynamic that what is true today may change. For instance, there are current debates in Great Britain and Switzerland for consideration of programs similar to that in place in Holland. In China, concern for the increasing size of the elderly population, as well as what seem to be inadequate government provisions for end-of-life health care are stimulating a strong movement for euthanasia—this despite the prevalence in that society of the Confucian tradition of respect for one's ancestors.[11] The outcome of these debates is the subject of much speculation, and given the increasing importance of China in the world's overall function, what evolves should be of major interest to the international community.

The Netherlands, Belgium, Luxembourg, and Colombia are clearly committed to a liberal approach toward euthanasia—active as well as passive. In other countries of the developed world, there currently are variances of laws in place, but yet substantial commonality exists between them.[12] Laws that govern active euthanasia or mercy killing are clear in most countries, and ignoring them can lead to an admission ticket to prison. Assisted suicide—whether by physician or otherwise—is another matter. Not surprisingly, in England, the birthplace of the hospice concept, palliative care is stressed, and there are specific laws that prohibit active and passive physician-assisted suicide and euthanasia. In fact, there has even been a recent attempt to prosecute Britons for merely helping their own family members to make the trip to Switzerland for the purpose of undergoing assisted suicide.[13] Not surprisingly, the court rejected the prosecution's attempt. In contrast, the liberal Swiss law makes it illegal for a person to assist in a suicide only when it is done for "selfish" reasons; otherwise, there are no limits on helping someone to die, and the "no limit" clause is almost all-inclusive. In fact, organizations—both for-profit and nonprofit—exist in Switzerland that make those very arrangements for citizens as well as for people from other countries. Seventy percent of those applying for the program are accepted. The reverse is true in Holland, in which two-thirds of the applicants for the euthanasia program are rejected on various grounds. Also in contrast to the liberal Swiss law, most countries allowing assisted suicide require the person to be terminally ill or demand that a doctor assist the death. In Germany, on the other hand, assisted suicide is legal, but with the caveat that the assistance is provided by family members or friends, since doctors are strictly prohibited by the German Medical Association from participating in the process. Terminally ill Germans, Britons, and others often go to Switzerland to end their lives.

Not surprisingly, there is considerable contention between the right-to-die activists and those more traditional Swiss who are appalled by what they view as a factory-like business of death. They are especially bothered by the influx of people from other countries who come specifically for assistance in dying. The Swiss organization Dignitas has helped more than 1,000 people die since 1998. Its founder, Ludwig Minelli, refutes critics of the organization's activities by comparing talk of prohibiting foreigners from coming to Switzerland to die to the country's decision to deny entry to Jews fleeing from the Holocaust during World War II. There are currently planned referenda designed to restrict and regulate such organizations, and by the time of the publication of this book, these practices may be altered or even prohibited.

I believe that a physician's participation in patient killing is a dance on a very precarious surface, whether active as in Holland and now in Luxembourg and Belgium, or passive as is permitted in Oregon, Washington State, or Montana. Even more certain in my mind is that the European practice, especially in Switzerland, in which nonphysicians are allowed to participate in another's suicide, is tantamount to the encouragement of mischief of the worst kind. At the risk of being thought cynical, I believe there is a dark side to human nature, and because of an unwillingness to assume goodness until it is demonstrated, I consider the slippery slope metaphor more than a catchy debating phrase. I believe it to be a predictable outcome. Throughout history, utopian ideals have disappointed more often than not.

There are those who suggest that the Dutch euthanasia experience should quell the fear of what might face America under a similar system. But it should be noted that some scholars do not consider this program to be functioning well. Even if these skeptics are in error, and even if their experience is mostly favorable, I believe it would be misleading to transpose the Dutch experience to the complex U.S. society. Holland is a small country with a fairly homogeneous population that is provided with universal health care coverage from birth to the grave. The latter fact makes potential financial motives for doctors at least theoretically somewhat less a factor in Holland. Other important differences between Holland and the United States do not bode well for the success of their euthanasia model in this country: The relationship between physicians and patients is different in Holland and, importantly, Dutch physicians do not labor under a cloud of legal threat, as is the case in the United States.

Despite all of this, it is worthwhile to take a closer look at the extended experience in Holland and objectively addresses the issues of active and passive euthanasia. The fact of the Dutch society being much smaller creates many differences from ours, one of which is a unique relationship between the patient and primary care physician. In Holland, the public relies on a neighborhood physician who usually lives in their midst and therefore has a much closer relationship with patients than American doctors do. That relationship should not be trivialized, because it is key to the functionality of the Dutch termination-of-life policy.

Because of the news value and sensationalism of the topic, one is inclined to think that active euthanasia is commonly practiced in Holland. Actually, the numbers are surprisingly small, and the overall frequency has changed only moderately in recent times. Since the inception of the practice, a steady increase of support by both public and physicians has occurred. In 1966, only 40 percent of the former was in favor of the practice; in 1988, that figure had risen to 81 percent; and by the year 2000, the public support for physician-assisted suicide or active euthanasia was 90 percent. Polling of Dutch physicians revealed that 57 percent have actually performed the procedure; another 30 percent said that if asked, they would, whereas only 10 percent of physicians said they would never do so. A 1995 report showed that a substantial majority of Dutch physicians consider the act, whether passive or active, to be part of their responsibility.[14] Whether this data reflects a modernization of society or merely a desensitization of both doctor and public is the subject of considerable debate. Dutch physicians choose to think of euthanasia as part of their job, while their critics view it as a devaluing of human life and a compromise of the medical profession. I would submit that just because a practice becomes more palatable doesn't mean that it is right. Isn't that what desensitization is all about? I am reminded of Aldous Huxley's 1932 futuristic novel, *Brave New World*,[15] which imagines a world possessed by a dehumanizing logic that is applied to the death process.

The Dutch process is fairly structured, and it is designed to disqualify all but a few patients from the program. First, a patient must request from the neighborhood doctor that his or her life be ended. All acceptable alternatives for relieving suffering should have been already suggested and tried, and the patient must feel that there is no other reasonable solution. Importantly, the patient must have a full plate of information. The physician must consult with a second and independent doctor who has examined the patient and who agrees. Finally, the primary care physician provides the service with a monitored standard of care. Most of the time, the patient administers the initial dose of the intravenous preparations, but if this fails, the attending physician "completes the job." In recent times, approximately 33,000 patients inquire about the process each year, and of these, almost 10,000 actually apply for candidacy. Over 65 percent are turned down because other means are available for relief or because one or more of the doctors involved felt that the underlying reason for the request was clinical depression.[16] In summary, if the patient requests it, a doctor can refuse and refer, can advice and arrange, or can actually administer the lethal potion designed to end life.

Of the 140,000 yearly deaths in Holland, 31 percent are from sudden and unexpected reasons; another 20 percent are allowed to die by withholding or withdrawing support systems; another 20 percent are terminally sedated; and about 4 percent undergo active euthanasia. Regarding this last percentage, in 1990, the figure was 2.9 percent, and by 2001, it had risen to 3.7 percent of all deaths. The causes for the requested termination of life have been consistent—most are for cancer-related issues, and 7–10 percent for cardiovascular or neurological reasons. Since pain is so effectively managed in this day and age, it alone is responsible for only a small percentage of requests for life termination procedures. Instead, it seems that the general avoidance of enduring the final stages of mental and physical deterioration is what motivates the majority of requests.[17]

It should be noted that even though the annual number of people whose lives are terminated in Holland by euthanasia has increased only moderately, there are current discussions in that country regarding the liberalization and expansion of the eligibility criteria to include Down syndrome and other birth defects associated with mental retardation. This suggests that insidious desensitization of the medical and lay public seems to be occurring. A friend of mine who is an extensively published and renowned bioethicist told me of his experiences at an international conference held in Europe this past year, in which he participated in a panel discussion that included several Dutch physicians. He privately asked one eminent scholar how it felt the first time he euthanized a patient in this government program. The physician confessed to very conflicted moral feelings. However, after performing a number of these acts, he was no longer bothered by participating in the process. The long-term data tends to show exactly that: The medical profession becomes desensitized to the act of killing.

Sissela Bok of the Harvard Center for Population and Developmental Studies has questioned the perception that the Dutch euthanasia experience is a success story.[18] According to Bok, there are growing concerns within Holland over abuse and slippage in the program. While active euthanasia is still technically illegal in Holland, it is tolerated; a physician is not prosecuted if it is shown that the government-dictated criteria have been strictly followed and the act has been promptly reported. Not surprisingly, the latter does not always happen. In fact, one report states that 59 percent of Dutch doctors admit they do not report their acts of euthanasia. Other worrisome data analysis shows that nearly 5 percent of all deaths in the Netherlands are caused by physicians, 25 percent of whom admitted that they had ended a patient's life without the patient's consent.[19] Inevitably, one problem begets another and authorities are thus unable to enforce the stringent and well-intended rules of the process. Furthermore, Bok says that 0.7 percent of those that were killed had not been competent to consent to the procedure and about half of those had never even expressed a desire for it—many were in a coma or demented. Finally, Bok's analysis reveals that in Holland, active euthanasia had been employed on severely disabled babies.[20]

Both Bok's analysis and the data of Kass are, however, vigorously contested.[21] Simply put, there are contradictory opinions and data regarding the Dutch program that are disturbing for those of us who look to summarizations and consensus for our education in certain matters. If Kass is correct, the actual number is uncertain. If such is not the case, even though there may be slippage and some suspicion of programmatic abuse in Holland, there does not seem to be a watershed of patients being rushed to termination. Whichever the case, it cannot be said that it could never happen if it hasn't already. Either version of the Dutch experience raises the question of the potential difficulty of holding the line against slippage of essential eligibility criteria. Whether this has actually happened in Holland is essentially irrelevant to America's social system; at most, it is of academic interest in American ethics circles. To think the Dutch euthanasia program would function as designed in the much larger and more complex American society is, in my opinion, an exercise in fantasy. It is worth noting again that the adoption of such a system is strongly opposed by the leadership of the American medical profession and many other leadership forces within the United States. While that may be an instinctively reactionary stance, it does in fact recognize how unrealistic the implementation of this "modern social concept" really is.

There have been numerous unsuccessful attempts to promote official programs for ending life other than those that succeeded in Oregon, Washington State, and Montana. Between 1991 and 2000, for instance, public referenda were held in California, Michigan, and Maine. Impressively, between the years of 1994 and 2007, there were twenty-one unsuccessful attempts by state legislatures to legalize euthanasia and/or assisted suicide. In each of the following states, there has been at least one attempt, and in others numerous attempts, to legislate such activities: Alaska, Arizona, California, Colorado, Connecticut, Hawaii, Illinois, Louisiana, Maine, Maryland, Massachusetts, Michigan, Mississippi, Nebraska, New Hampshire, New Mexico, New York, Rhode Island, Vermont, and Wisconsin. Eight states—Iowa, Louisiana, Maryland, Michigan, Rhode Island, South Carolina, New York State, and Virginia have actually passed laws prohibiting assisted suicide.[22] In the case of New York State, a 1994 Task Force on Life and the Law studied the issues of assisted suicide and euthanasia as it pertained to medical practice in the state.

To the credit of its members, the Task Force recommended the continuation of the existing ban on physician-assisted suicide. Their opposition to lifting it was based on the grounds that "legalizing such an act would be unwise and dangerous public policy because of several social risks: no matter how carefully guidelines are drawn, assisted suicide would be practiced the way other medicine in the United States is, that is, through the prism of social inequality and bias."[23] Furthermore, the Task Force concluded that minorities, the poor, and the elderly would be at greatest risks for abuse. Additionally, the group predicted that financial imperatives might usurp guidelines as doctors, hospitals, insurers, and governments all seek to save money. This was an important recognition of a system's vulnerability to the frailty of human restraint. It would be wonderful if humankind stayed on the straight and narrow, but the New York State commission apparently realistically did not believe this would be the case.

I have combined the various subdivisions of euthanasia in this discussion, so that my reasoning weaves in and out of the discussions of both active and passive physician-assisted suicide. Since the latter is already legal in three states in this country and, according to the data in the preceding paragraph, there will almost certainly be other movements to legalize physician-assisted suicide in the future, I want to be clear in stating my belief that they are equally dangerous to our system of social values and equally compromising to the integrity of the medical profession. Make no mistake, the "Slippery Slope" theory is far more than theoretical, and my use of the uppercase in reference to it reflects the fact that it has been a named part of the debate for over a century.

Some critics of this theory have likened its purveyors to a doomsday cult that repeatedly predicts the end of the world, only for followers to discover the next day that things are pretty much as they were. The debate over the Slippery Slope theory is ongoing and rigorous, but much of my personal endorsement of it is predicated on my slightly dark view of human nature. I disavow any doomsday scenarios for humanity; however, it's hard to ignore the numerous historical precedents that have lined up to create perfect conditions for human misadventure. My lack of confidence in human beings' inherent goodness is not born of a religious conviction, and I do not believe that man was born in original sin. For those that do, I mean no confrontation by this revelation of a personal belief; I only seek to eliminate that birthright as the basis of my skepticism regarding human capabilities. In other words, I don't know if humans are inherently bad or not, but I do know that on a fairly consistent basis they are corruptible.

In planning the writing of this book, I had no idea that my research would lead me so extensively into the matter of euthanasia. The more I studied the history of this and related matters, however, the more I became impressed with the dangers that would accompany the legalization of killing, both by doctors as well as others, and the more I realized that left unchecked the world of cancer medicine would be dramatically affected. To deny the Slippery Slope argument is to ignore the reality of what has been done historically by civilized people in developed countries. I have discussed how in Germany a wave of activism in a social environment of silent collusion combined to fertilize a financial imperative for thinning the population of the vulnerable, which to me should be called euthanasia of social convenience. At first blush, one might think that the German experience was a "Nazi thing," but clearly, the notion was rampant before the advent of the National Socialist Party came along. Was that period in the Weimar Republic not a buildup—a desensitizing—a conditioning—to what was made official policy in 1939? Was there not a slippery slope at work in all of this? I would submit that the average German of the twentieth century was no less moral than we are, and I would further argue that under the proper circumstances, we are vulnerable to much of the same social poison that brought them to amorality. The dire financial situation in post–World War I Germany in large part spawned the need for rationing of important resources, and hence the euthanasia movement. There was, essentially, an economic imperative in place. In the United States, we have been blessed with continued wealth; however, that could change, and conceivably to the point where health care would be strictly rationed. I leave the potential scenario to the imagination of the reader, upon whom I urge realistic thinking in avoiding naïveté about the fundamental goodness of human beings.

This Slippery Slope theory is not the only argument against legalization of physician involvement in the induction of patient death. Throughout Judeo-Christian and Eastern religious philosophy, there is an intrinsic wrongness associated with killing, and the blatant performance of this act surely invites concern for the integrity of the profession. This part of the Oath is clear and should stand. When physicians become killers, rather than healers, can patients really trust them to advise and to do what is in their best interest? Is a physician not vulnerable to pressures from a system that is run by decision makers who function at a higher bureaucratic level—an impersonal place where decisions on distribution of resources are decided on the basis of flow charts and computer projections? We don't have to look any further than contemporary corporate organizations that actually presume to grade their doctor employees, in large measure judging their value on the basis of how many patients per hour they grind through the system. Does anyone doubt the fact that in modern urban hospital systems there is now and will be more intense pressure on physicians, financial incentives against expensive treatments, and a devaluing of interpersonal relationships between physicians and patients? Does anyone doubt that such a set of guidelines can potentially have a substantial impact on a physician's judgment and decision-making process? If a physician's integrity is not implicitly trusted to function on behalf of the patient, will any patient be able to relax? These issues, all of which are either directly or indirectly financial, will only increase in the future as we grapple with a system that is currently in considerable turmoil. To drive this point home, consider, for example, that in New York City, 25 percent of the citizens have no health care insurance. If and when health care rationing becomes a reality, is it not predictable that there would be financial incentives created to end life, especially if the process has been legalized?

The possibilities become even more corrupted when hard-core personal questions are posed. Does anyone doubt that there could be pressures imposed on a doctor from greedy and impatient family members to encourage termination of the life of a chronically ill or demented parent who is inconveniently and resiliently clinging to life? Does anyone doubt that some physicians could be influenced by financial incentives in such a situation? Physicians should be and usually are honorable, but greed and avarice are not limited to individuals outside the medical profession.

Some argue that the autonomy of patients gives them the right and the ability to protect themselves and determine their own fate. I submit that this point of view is illusory. A trusted physician possesses considerable influence and power over a chronically ill patient, especially if, as is so often the case, that patient already feels like a burden to others or, as is also so often the case, is clinically depressed. Might there develop a subset of elderly who feel a "duty to die"? Furthermore, what if that same guilt-ridden patient is under the influence of medication? Consider also the circumstances of those patients who suffer dementia, a touch of paranoia, or have a limited capacity to comprehend; imagine their vulnerability to persuasion. Finally, consider such a patient's dilemma when legal guardianship is within the dominion of someone lacking in fiduciary integrity. Within the context of a euthanasia discussion, do any of these remotely resemble real autonomy? I think not!

I have already cited the Dutch experience, in which a number of patients put to death never asked for it, and some others were not even awake to be consulted. To paraphrase Battin, in a society in which it is legal to terminate life, or in which it is legal to assist in patient suicide, the vulnerable could be socially programmed to think of themselves as unworthy to remain alive.[24] This notion of an elderly person feeling an obligation to die is not without historic example. Some Native American groups had in place a social system in which older persons, upon feeling that they could not carry their share of the work, would order their oldest son to kill them or would go off to die on their own.. My point is simply that the complexity of psychiatric forces that affect the thinking and attitudes of the elderly can be compelling, and under the right legal and social circumstances, the "obligation to die" is more than a random theoretical possibility.

Thus, under an "ideal" scenario, the elderly, the chronically ill, and others would be protected only by unenforceable guidelines that have been set up by well-meaning utopian theoreticians. That we must even consider these sinister possibilities is an ugly necessity—shame on human nature, but welcome to the real world! In the words of Niccolo Machiavelli, one of history's most committed realists, "it seemed more suitable to me to search after the effectual truth of the matter rather than an imagined one . . . for there is such a gap between how one lives and how one ought to live that anyone who abandons what is done for what ought to be done learns his ruin rather than his preservation."[25]

Let's be clear, physicians have been helping people die since antiquity, and even in the stern vocabulary of Roman Catholic doctrine, the principle of double effect, if followed explicitly, allows flexibility. While death must never be intentionally caused, the physician may licitly use drugs for the control of pain and relief of agony, even though foreseeing, though not intending, that this might cause an earlier death. Although this is generally considered Catholic doctrine, it has been widely embraced by the secular segment of society and the profession, and because of its widespread applicability, I include the basic criteria of the principle, although a discussion of each is beyond the scope of this writing. As defined, one may perform an action that is intended to achieve a good effect if it is foreseen that a negative effect will also result; that is to say, the principle of double effect governs situations in which one action is followed by two effects—one good and intended, and the other negative, and even though unintended, foreseen.

The four main conditions that govern this fundamental ethical principle are: (1) the action in itself is good or at least indifferent, that is, neither good nor bad; (2) the good effect and not the bad effect is intended; (3) the good effect is not produced by means of the bad effect; and (4) there is a proportionately grave reason for permitting the bad effect—the bad effect must not exceed the good. When strictly followed, the practical ramifications of this principle are profound. For example, removing a cancerous uterus from a pregnant woman produces a tragic effect for the child, but assuming there is no other less harmful option, the act is good, although the death of the child is not.

Through the strictly followed guidelines of the principle of double effect, the concept of terminal sedation becomes workable. It is not meant to include a directly intended overdose; instead, the term *terminal sedation* can only be included within this principle when the intent of sedation is to relieve pain and suffering, while knowing the sedation may depress other bodily functions such as respiration, which may in turn lead to pneumonia and an earlier death. Essentially, between modern pain control methods and terminal sedation, the trajectory to death can be made less formidable. Even though some linguistic perfectionists argue that the principle of double effect is merely a matter of semantics designed to provide a means of assuaging the blisters of conscience, I believe it to be a practical and ethical tool when seeking functionality with a problem faced daily by many of the medical profession. Beyond that, I leave the defense of the doctrine to scholars of ethics and theology.

Finally, mention should be made of a unique corollary to the matter of physician involvement with patient death. Occasionally, a medically fragile patient develops a cancer that ideally would require a substantial operation; however, given the patient's poor health, the operative mortality would be unacceptably high. Given these circumstances, any wise surgeon advises other avenues of treatment, or perhaps nothing, save palliation. However, there are some patients who don't accept this, and who attempt to force an operation— thinking that if they are otherwise destined to die, they may as well "go for it" and die on the operating table. On several occasions in my surgical career, I have had such a patient attempt to persuade me to operate, despite my warning that such an endeavor would almost certainly end in death. Even though I have always understood the fatalistic logic of these patients, I have never succumbed to the pressure to practice what I considered to be bad medicine, and to engage in, by my standards, an unethical act. While it is understandable, it's audacious and inconsiderate for a patient or a family to ask this of a surgical team. Merely asking a surgeon to participate in such a charade reveals ignorance of the seriousness and sense of responsibility that most substantive surgeons and anesthesiologists bring to their job. Honoring such a request would in effect constitute a form of physician-assisted suicide—the very same that has been under discussion in the previous paragraphs, and which I consider to be unethical.

It should be noted that many surgeons have faced an inherently very dangerous operation and after the good and the potential bad are weighed they have chosen to operate. Such a circumstance is not rare in cardiovascular and neurological surgery, although is less common in cancer surgery. But this circumstance is not the same as the extreme case in which the surgery would almost certainly exceed the tolerance of a particular patient.

Losing a patient on the operating table—whether expected or otherwise—is a monumental event, and a surgeon who has experienced it never forgets. Vivid in my memory is an unanticipated operative death thirty years ago of a three-year-old patient that resulted from factors out of my control.

Illogically, I still wonder if the patient would have survived had I been wiser and more skillful. I have talked to other surgeons who have similar retained memories of operating room misfortune.

When one considers the methods with which physicians can help in the process of death, and when the wonderful work of the hospice systems is added to the mix, it is a testimony to the intellectual fastidiousness of those who continue to seek clarification and definition. I suspect that the search for both will go on for some time, and I might add that it is appropriate for this to happen. In the meantime, however, life and death go on and the practicing physicians must continue to deal with both. The evolving data on the functionality of physicians in this regard suggests that we are keeping pace with our changing societal behavior. Two studies in particular focus on this trend: In a 1989 investigation, over 85 percent of critical care physicians admitted to withholding or withdrawing life sustaining treatments in patients with irreversible or terminal disease.[26] In a more contemporary comparative study done in 1997, two time periods—1987–1988, and 1992–1993—were analyzed and the rate of withholding and withdrawing life sustenance in the terminally ill went from 51 percent in the former to 90 percent in the latter.[27] Other data substantiates this method of dealing with the process of dying. For example, in the United States, approximately 80 percent of deaths occur in hospitals or some other nursing facility, and of those, 70 percent have had the elective withholding of some life-sustaining treatment. In this country 1.3 million deaths per year occur after withholding or withdrawal of such equipment.[28]

All of these data have to be looked at with some scientific skepticism, since it depends on the performance and admission of once unmentionable acts. It follows that any inaccuracies would be on the low side—that is, the percentage may actually be higher. It is a fact that many physicians receive requests from patients for physician-assisted suicide or even more direct intervention, and one realistically has to assume that some of these requests are granted. It is impossible to know how often this happens, since it occurs outside of the law. One can only imagine that throughout history, many well-connected and influential figures have requested and received physician as-sistance—both active and passive—in making the passage from life to death. As a means of sparking curiosity in this matter, the reader is asked to imagine the mathematical improbability of two of the most famous Founders—Jefferson and Adams—dying within hours of each other on July 4, 1826—the fiftieth anniversary of the signing of the Declaration of Independence—that single day in history that best exemplifies their commonality of purpose. Coincidence? Perhaps.

· 11 ·

Suicide: Patient Conceived, Planned, and Consummated

The thought of suicide is a great consolation: by means of it one gets successfully through many a bad night.

—*Friedrich Wilhelm Nietzsche (1844–1900)*

*O*bviously, suicide does not require physician assistance. Up to this point, I have interwoven the discussions of physician-assisted suicide with active euthanasia. In this chapter, however, all types of euthanasia will be excluded from the discussion, and I will focus on the act in the context in which it is usually spontaneously committed.

Much of the information regarding suicide throughout the world is neither well reported nor well collated; hence, misinformation is to be expected. Furthermore, because of cultural eccentricities, the global suicide burden can only be estimated. Data sets are undoubtedly distorted in India, for instance, where suicide is actually illegal, and the aftermath of the act impacts on the surviving family; in fact, the law there is thought to be responsible for a tenfold underestimate of self-inflicted death.[1] In China, where 30 percent of suicides in the world occur, a three to one rural prevalence of its occurrence explains why many such deaths are unreported.[2] It is thought that approximately 300,000 suicides occur each year in China, as opposed to the 31,000 in the United States.[3] Even factoring in the different sizes of the two countries, the difference is striking. The World Health Organization estimates that throughout the world, there are one million self-inflicted deaths per year.[4] This figure represents approximately a 1.5 percent of all deaths—a number that makes suicide the tenth leading cause of death worldwide.[5] Undoubtedly, these are grossly underestimated numbers. In China as many as 15 percent of all deaths probably go unreported, and one is only left to speculate how little administrative attention is paid to determining what is suicide and what is not. Such embedded data is not limited to Asia; a number of Western countries such as France, several Scandinavian countries, and others have policies in which suicides are not consistently separated from deaths of "unknown" cause. This practice of combining data to record deaths almost certainly alters the true suicide rate that is reported to the World Health Organization.

Despite these statistical limitations, there are some consistent facts worthy of noting: Rates vary greatly, with the greatest burden in developing countries; throughout the world, men are substantially more likely than women to commit suicide; and the overall suicide rate in the elderly seems to be diminishing while during the last fifty years that rate has increased substantially in the younger generations.

Certain contributory factors afford some help in risk-factor development: acute psychosocial crises, psychiatric disorders, pessimism or hopelessness, impulsivity, family history, certain childhood factors—all are associated with a higher overall suicide rate. The most important factor that applies to suicide in both cancer patients and others is that the completed suicide rate associated with depression is many times the general population risk. In fact, the numbers are staggering: more than 50 percent of all people who die by suicide are depressed.[6] If one looks at the data from the opposite direction, approximately 4 percent of clinically depressed individuals die by suicide, a number that is even higher in males. Importantly, of those individuals afflicted with bipolar disorders, 10–15 percent die by suicide.[7] Other factors: white Americans over African Americans and Hispanics, both male and female homosexuals over heterosexuals, drug and alcohol dependents, and individuals who have suffered physical and sexual abuse during childhood all reflect a higher suicide rate than the controls in each respective group. A final daunting statistic is that in 40 percent of suicides, there has been a previous suicide attempt.[8] In fact, this last risk factor stands out among all others.

With regard to the older population, if one excludes mental illness and looks only at matters that contribute to suicide, three of life's problems stand out as constituting risk factors—physical illness, interpersonal problems, and bereavement. Since this book mostly concerns matters pertaining to cancer, let us look at the first. In an important paper, Harwood and colleagues reported that in fully two-thirds of the older suicide victims studied, physical illness contributed to the suicide.[9] A similar study of North American older suicide victims and also a study focused on their Scandinavian counterparts both suggest that physical illnesses—especially malignant and neurological disorders—are associated with a particularly high suicide rate in the elderly.[10] Not a small complicating issue in the evaluation of all of these data is the fact that the link between suicide and physical illness, including cancer, may be mediated through depressive symptoms. According to Harwood et al., of those in whom physical illness was thought to be an impetus for their suicide, 60 percent also suffered from depression during the months before the act.[11] While it's a foregone conclusion for psychiatrists, for those of us lacking sophistication in this arena, this information serves to reaffirm the fact that depression is not limited to people with mental illness.

All of this data leads to one of the themes of this book—caring for cancer patients is a uniquely challenging endeavor, and in addition to all of the other risk considerations, the cancer patient is more likely to commit suicide compared to age- and gender-matched cohorts.[12] On a number of occasions, cancer patients have approached me with "the possibility" of suicide—some with a sense of desperation, and others coolly, as if conducting an intellectual exercise. Such probing most likely reflects an underlying thought process referred to in psychiatric jargon as suicidal ideations. These queries—whether obtuse or direct—ought not shock cancer doctors or deter them from counseling the patient in a realistic and mature manner. Most psychiatric literature suggests that the incidence of suicide ideations—though a significant precursor to the actual act of suicide—is substantially more frequent than completed suicide; the latter does not necessarily follow the former. In reviewing a number of studies regarding this matter, one is struck by the complexity of the issues and with the lack of reliability of controlled data. Translating suicidal ideations into predictive data is tricky business. For example, a substantial percentage of college-age individuals have thought about committing suicide. In addition to this phenomenon, if one considers the prevalence of mental illness, especially depression, both bipolar and otherwise the influences of drugs and alcohol and, finally, the whole subculture of patients dying with physician assistance (i.e., terminal sedation), even experts on these matters must often rely on estimates. Despite these flawed methods, many valuable conclusions regarding the relative risk-factor profile have been developed for the various types of suicide. This text is primarily devoted to cancer-related matters, but in order to understand this subset of the suicide population, the reader should first consider suicide generically.

It is important to recognize that the oncologist is often the patient's first outlet for his or her most intimate thoughts; therefore, when suicidal ideations surface, no matter how subtly verbalized, the physician should respond by encouraging, rather than discouraging, dialogue with the patient. Lest oncologists underrate the importance of this moment in time, I draw attention to the fact that a substantial number of cancer patients who commit suicide visit their cancer physician in the last month of their life.[13] The state of alertness to the likelihood of suicide should be heightened even more in individuals with malignancies of certain select organ sites—breast, prostate, and head and neck cancers all seem to be associated with higher rates of suicide than other sites.[14] The patient's "overture"—no matter how subtle—represents an important juncture, essentially, a reaching out for help. From this point on, the oncologist must uncouple morality and suicide and react as a physician, rather than a theologian. In my opinion, it's dismissive and condescending to respond to such a trial balloon with triteness: "it's not a good idea," "it's morally wrong," "that won't solve anything." And most unforgivable is to avoid the discussion altogether. Following such a nonproductive visit with the physician, a cancer patient is left with the same questions, the same motivations, and the same sense of desperation that he or she came in with. The major change that results from such psychiatric myopia is that the physician has largely lost the confidence of the patient and has probably squandered any hope of influencing the course of events. One of the early lessons in psychiatric training is to never underestimate the significance of a patient talking about suicide, no matter how innocent sounding. While not always a prologue to action, it must always be taken seriously.

On several occasions, I have had the sad experience of patients actually taking their own life, and even though I recognized the rationale, each evoked within me a sense of having failed in my leadership and guidance of a desperate patient. After the fact, I pondered whether if I had established the correct relationship with the patient or perhaps picked up on certain signals, this might not have happened. For the compulsive, the sense of failed responsibility is like the memory of an odor—amorphous and pervasive. On the other hand, I am conflicted by my ambivalence in this matter. Vivid recollections of a number of patients linger within me, but two in particular reverberate in my memory. Each was dying of refractory head and neck cancer that was creating unspeakable misery and degradation—odor, drooling, pain, embarrassment. When they ended their own lives I felt relief; at a minimum, I understood their reasons. This confession may be good for my psyche, but forgetting is another matter.

It is intuitive to me that the mandate for alertness relative to suicide prevention should be more intense in patients with favorable situations and can ethically be looked at with different standards than patients like the ones I just cited with refractory head and neck cancer. Regarding the attention given to those with favorable prognoses, it is important to note that the prevalence of suicide is probably highest in the first three months following diagnosis of cancer, and then peaks again at about one year after treatment.[15] Additionally, there are data suggesting that, for unexplained reasons, the risk for adult survivors of childhood cancer is elevated over noncancer patients.[16] More understandable is that the risk factor for suicide in cancer patients is higher in the elderly. Finally, we cannot loose sight of the threefold increase in suicide rate among cancer-afflicted widowed men compared with those who are married.[17]

The take-home message here is that in dealing with this matter, the oncologist should individualize the situation and tailor the response by considering the risk factors and characteristics that have been referred to in the preceding paragraphs. Of course, all of these machinations are considerations within the activities of the psycho-oncologist's consultations and care. At another point in this book, I state that psychological support given to the cancer patient should be delivered circumferentially—from all members of the team, but especially from the oncologist to whom the patient extended the overture. Essentially, that team member has a greater responsibility in the process by virtue of the fact that the patient apparently feels a stronger connection to that person.

One cannot avoid discussing the matter of physician assistance in suicide, and in this regard, oncologists and anyone else seeking to care for cancer patients must have their standards clearly established. The alertness of a cancer physician to the patient's signals differs from the less subtle circumstance in which a patient actively seeks help in ending his or her life. No matter how heart-wrenching a patient's misery or how compelling the appeals from the patient or family, a physician's active involvement in a suicide is prohibited by law, except in Oregon, Washington State, and Montana. To step outside of legal restrictions is foolish and irresponsible. I speak of this with no moral overtone whatsoever—it's simply not permitted. How a physician personally feels about it or how much one might disagree with the restrictions on one's freedom to respond to these desperate requests are both irrelevant issues. In the final analysis, such active involvement is in violation of the law except in three states.

Even when trying to make a statement of principle, for a physician to ignore the law is foolhardy. Once again, I point to the incarceration of Doctor Jack Kevorkian for what he thought to be justified. While the cultlike support he enjoyed in his heyday continues to some degree, his story has been a valuable lesson in self-destructive behavior. So when a patient asks about suicide, physician involvement must be limited to conversation and advice only. Recently, a grand jury in Atlanta, Georgia, indicted four members of a suicide assistance group for their actions. The upcoming litigation should help define the future of other nonmedical organizations, such as the Final Exit Network, the Hemlock Society, and others that advise people with terminal diseases about suicide. My attitude about such organizations is that while we should avoid being judgmental, the medical profession should have no official connection with them and should abstain from expressing opinions on their activities.

In the past, I've dealt with suicide queries from doomed patients in a variety of ways, but the theme common to my response has always involved the reassurance that I would be available until the end, and that I would exercise a very liberal use of medications for sedation and pain. Regarding this latter statement, the concept of terminal sedation is introduced, and the patient is allowed to rely on anything short of outright overdosing. The physician must keep in mind the consistent fear that is common to most cancer patients of being abandoned by their doctor or their family. Since terminal sedation is within our legal and ethical capabilities if the criteria are followed, and since today's pain control is so effective, physicians are able to mitigate the agony of cancer-related terminal life more than ever before. It is important to note, however, that pain alone does not frequently explain the motivation to end one's life. In fact, there is survey data from the Dutch experience that shows pain is responsible for only 5 percent of the inquiries about that country's euthanasia program. The same is probably true among those who consider suicide in the United States. The motivation is usually not singular, but instead amorphous and broad based. Consider, if you will, that the enormity of what the cancer patient faces—the forces of depression/anxiety, discouragement, fear, concern for financial and family compromise, a desperate concern for privacy and dignity, and lastly the avoidance of going through the general misery of the terminal period—all come together in an avalanche of psychic and physical forces. Some patients simply say to themselves, "Who needs all of this?"

Depression alone is an insidious but powerful enemy that can emotionally consume a terminal cancer patient, and often it is accompanied by anxiety. Fifteen to twenty-five percent of cancer patients are affected substantially by depression.[18] That relentless partner of depression—anxiety—has been studied both independently and together with the former. Depression and panic attacks seem to be more prevalent in the younger population. This association tends to decline with age, so the elderly handle the situation better.[19] If unrelenting pain is thrown into the mix, the perfect psychiatric circumstances exist to overwhelm a cancer patient. I think of this as a circle of torment that feeds itself—depression and anxiety enhanced by pain, which leads to a sense of hopelessness and deeper depression, and so on. Even in the noncancer patient, the duality of depression and anxiety occurs. One can only imagine how much more intense the syndrome is when the fear of cancer and death enter the picture. Both antidepressants and antianxiety medications have come of age, however, and, especially in the patient destined to die of cancer, when this new pharmacopoeia is combined with proper pain management, the all-important involvement of a psycho-oncologist, and the diligence and staying power of the alpha oncologist, the terminal phase of the disease is dramatically improved over previous times. In my experience, a majority of cancer patients who have suicidal thoughts ultimately decide against it when the "the circle of torment" is treated and the alpha oncologist has engaged in forthright dialogue about the subject. Having said this, I should point out that until relatively recently, cancer physicians and even cancer teams have not done a very good job in dealing with this syndrome of depression, pain, and anxiety. Fortunately, as the concept of the functional cancer team matures, we are getting better at it.

Most patients abhor the thought of committing suicide, many for religious reasons. It is fundamental to Judeo-Christian, Islamic, and Hindu theology that death should come at God's will, rather than one's own. These philosophies teach that life is a gift from God and to arbitrarily end it usurps the power of the creator. Those that follow these tenets feel that the will of God with respect to this matter must be taken on faith. It follows, then, that since killing is intrinsically wrong and suicide is self-killing, to commit suicide is wrong. It's an extraordinary contradiction that jihadists in the news today justify suicide bombing by religious authority despite the fact that the Holy Koran does not condone suicide. Roman Catholic traditions are based on specific doctrine that not only condemns the actual act of suicide but also considers it wrong for someone to aid in the act of another's suicide. In fact, in Roman Catholic history, the most stringent of interpretations of the transgression of suicide prevented persons who have taken their own lives from being embraced in the after-death rituals of the Church. Modern adaptation does grant the concession that those who have committed suicide are often emotionally disturbed and not in possession of full reason; therefore, contemporary practice usually allows full ritual performance. Until this recent flexibility of the Church's previous attitude, this was an area of some sensitivity and resentment among those Catholics who are family members of suicide victims. But basically, despite this modification, the Church has been consistent in its teachings since suicide was formally banned in the sixth century. Other religious philosophies—Jewish and Christian alike—are more lenient and tolerant in dealing with this issue than is Roman Catholic orthodoxy.

In addition to the religion-based objections to suicide, other arguments for its wrongness are used—especially those that relate to the emotional impact of the act on the family, friends, and colleagues left behind. Not infrequently there is an enormous effect following suicide, and the long-term physic influences can be especially harmful to young children.[20]

It seems intuitive that suicide among cancer victims should be classified and thought of differently from those without cancer. There is often a sense of inevitability and the dread of tangible suffering while a killer lurks, and even in those who are emotionally sound prior to the development of their cancer, the compounding effects of depression and anxiety frequently emerge. On the other hand, the noncancer-related suicide is a different and perhaps sadder matter—another topic for another book that is composed by an expert in these matters. These are topics of profound importance to psychiatrists, and the management of patients who suffer from clinical depression, drug dependency, and other discouraging problems present challenges unique in medicine, although obviously such mental illnesses are not mutually exclusive from the emotional burdens of the cancer patient. But at the risk of over-simplifying a complex topic, these psychodynamics that lead to suicide are generally different from those of cancer patients. In cancer patients the psychiatrist seems to face three separate forces, albeit blended together: first, the patient's fear of dealing with a relentless downhill journey to death; secondly, an organic depression-anxiety syndrome that is often present; and finally, fear of the unknown, of nothingness, and in many individuals, fear of the end of existence.

The reader should be clear that I am not advocating that oncologists attempt to manage the suicidal thoughts and inclinations of cancer patients. However, neither should they shy away from engaging the patient in an unflinching dialogue. Psychiatric consultation and management is vital to the modern cancer team, but the process starts with a mature cancer physician who is not intimidated by the suicide word; and importantly, the psychological involvement of the oncologist taking care of the cancer is in no way mutually exclusive from that of the psycho-oncologist. Even while the psychiatrist is doing what he or she does, there should be no prohibition of the oncologist to engage in intimate conversation with the patient. At a minimum, simply talking about suicide gives a doomed cancer patient the reassurance of autonomy, that is, jurisdiction over his or her body—something that may in itself have therapeutic value. The Nietzsche quotation at the outset of this chapter suggests exactly this, and seems to me to provide an imperative for the alert and mature cancer physician to encourage and engage, rather than discourage a suicide dialogue when a patient brings the matter up.

As is stated on several occasions in this book, a vulnerable cancer patient's reliance on their oncologist can be extraordinary, and it is not unusual for the patient to look to that physician for advice and counsel on a variety of health-related matters—psychiatry, nutrition, their aunt's migraines—you get the picture. The role of the "perceived expert" on all matters medical must be handled with tact, realism, humility, and always with graciousness and generosity. It's a simple thing to disavow expertise while also showing obvious interest by offering suggestions on some questions and by promoting appropriate referrals when indicated. In this day and age of super-specialization, it is important to remind ourselves that we are still physicians and we should still attempt to look after and care for the "whole patient."

It is worth noting that throughout history other cultures have looked at suicide differently; and even in the United States today, there is reasonable support for the individual's right to decide when and how death should come. So after all of the considerations, we are left to deal on a practical level with a segment of the population who face the finality of uncontrolled cancer, who are unencumbered either by religious inhibitions or family matters, who are not worried about the afterlife, and who do not wish to be terminally sedated lest they lose the ability to alertly deal with their own demise. When such a patient says to me, "I want to be in control of my own death"—a statement that I view as meaning a desire for autonomy—I respond, "Even though I can't help you do the deed, you have my understanding and best wishes for whatever awaits you." This statement is not an advocacy, but merely an articulation of my belief that a person not restricted by those factors that I have mentioned should indeed have control over their own destiny. The stoic philosophy of life and death of the ancient Greek philosophers[21] promoted the notion that a person should be responsible for the timing and character of his or her death. And later, the Romans espoused and even encouraged suicide. Mind you, *I do not* advocate this somewhat cynical view of the exiting of life; but in this writing, I seek to defend the right of those that do.

II

INTERACTING WITH CANCER PATIENTS AND THEIR FAMILIES

· *12* ·

Informal Physician-Patient Communication

Over the years, I have been regaled with stories of "the cancer experience" from friends, friends of friends, family, patients, and even strangers who approached me after seeing and being cared for by other doctors. This often occurs at social gatherings, which provide an interface between the nonmedical and medical worlds. Often the influence of the party spirit emboldens people to discuss personal and family medical experiences, occasionally at great length, and also to ask for opinions about ongoing personal medical issues. While some physicians feel this intrusion to be a breach of their privacy and are annoyed, most understand, are good listeners, and accept it as coming with the territory. I admit that I have always been slightly flattered by this process, and while I try not to encourage it, I listen and reply, being very careful not to say anything that undermines or contradicts previously given medical advice. In the case of them having gotten obviously wrong recommendations, at most I will say that if they are not confident or trusting of their medical team, they should seek other opinions. People are usually clever in reading between the lines.

We in the profession should always keep in mind that medical topics are usually interesting to the lay public, and especially for scientifically oriented people, whether they be in the profession or not. Many such issues provide fertile ground for social dialogue when unacquainted people are searching for ways to connect. People often think of physicians as outliers in a crowd, and because laypeople sometimes are at a loss for words on such occasions, they enter this zone of conversation out of nervousness—thinking that a physician likes to talk about medicine. When the approach is based on the hypothetical rather than on the personal, then it seems to me to be equivalent to any other scientific topic, such as the space shuttle, or solar energy. The personal discussions are the ones that are tricky.

101

Listening and giving advice to people who seek an unofficial appraisal of how they are doing and how their treating team is performing can be an extraordinarily sensitive matter. It's easy to judge another physician's performance when one does not have the responsibility of making decisions that can be life-or-death matters. By and large, these unofficial consultations are usually sought in social settings, and what I try to provide under these circumstances is the role of an interpreter, an explainer, if you will, of what they have been told and what they understand or have failed to understand. It is really important for the casual advisor not to undermine the patient's confidence in their medical team.

I take issue with some physicians' sense of violation of their privacy when people approach them in social settings. To practice medicine is to be a public servant, and the potential for such intrusions is at the core of the lifestyle. No matter how the "cornered" physician might feel, it is ill mannered to brush the person aside. There is almost always some element of embarrassment on the part of the person approaching a physician under these circumstances, and a dismissive or arrogant attitude leaves a social wound that creates bad public relations for the profession; and the last thing we need is bad PR.

Regarding the imagery of the profession, I have always thought doctors ought to serve as ambassadors for medicine, because the lay public is often ambivalent, and not infrequently antagonistic, about us. While they may still respect and hold the profession in esteem, much of the affection that previously existed has been lost in recent times. Perhaps the fact that we thrive off the misfortune of others renders the profession vulnerable to public resentment; however, I hope that sentiment is not rampant, and I would prefer to seek a less cynical explanation. Obviously, these huge generalities don't apply universally, and a negative attitude toward the profession varies from one community to another and from one geographic area of the country to another. That it does exist at all, however, should be of real concern to all physicians, because so much of what we do, especially in the cancer arena, is a high-stakes attempt to salvage life, and our endeavors in that regard require dependence, trust, and courage on the part of the patient. A variety of the forces of modern society have taken some of the sweetness out of our daily lives and, when combined with the extraordinary current state of turmoil in the medical profession, there should be little wonder that there are a number of unhappy physicians and patients as well. Part of the mission of this book is to discuss the partial rectification of this state by means of emphasizing the positive values of a more respectful time—more respectful for patient and physician alike. From a layman's perspective, mending must involve the public realization that doctors are, by and large, mostly good people who are truly concerned about a patient's welfare. While some are arrogant and insensitive, most are not.

It is my hope that young doctors will accept the responsibility of being goodwill ambassadors for the profession. The physician-patient social encounter that I refer to above is an example of an opportunity to do just that. In being cornered at a social gathering, extricating oneself while seeming interested and concerned usually does not require wizardry but only conversational and communicative skills and common courtesy. My advice to doctors is to avoid personal medical conversations at social gatherings when possible, but if cornered, be gracious. My advice to patients is to understand that to corner a doctor socially is often inappropriate, and in general, one should avoid doing it. When a physician gets involved in such a medical discussion, he or she should be mindful that the more life-threatening the topic, the more sensitive and delicate is the physician's part of the conversation. It follows then, when cancer is being discussed, there is usually a much more sober undercurrent in the patient's demeanor.

In an effort to look at all sides of this subtopic, we should all be reminded that many doctors do not excel at small talk, and in an effort to fill in the gaps, are more than willing to talk at length about what is familiar to them. Why a layperson should be skeptical of the doctor who is willing to "talk medicine" at length has some bearing on the subject of the next chapter.

· 13 ·

Patient Confidentiality and Special Patient Circumstances

$\mathcal{T}$he physician who is loose with patient confidences is in violation of a sacred trust. This is true for all medical confidences, but with cancer, it is monumental in importance. The Oath to which I have eluded is very clear and uncompromising regarding a patient's right to total privacy; the absoluteness of this commandment is never in doubt. Anyone hearing a doctor chatting about identifiable medical information should be wary of trusting such a marginally ethical individual, who at best has questionable judgment. In these litigious times, loose-lipped professionals will be held accountable for their indiscretions. During World War II when espionage was rampart, posters were hung throughout Great Britain that read, "Loose Lips Sink Ships." One might apply that same caution to health care professionals, especially physicians. Loose lips can sink careers.

I recall an unhappy story involving a breach of confidentiality and an unfortunate turn of events for a young doctor. When I was in training at Barnes Hospital in St. Louis, a resident in another specialty was fired after a less-than-discrete discussion with another resident while riding on a hospital elevator. He was talking in a low but clear voice about how one of his patient's alcoholism was complicating his care. It happened that one of the patient's adult children had just arrived from out of town, and yes, was on that same elevator, at exactly the same time. As it turned out, the patient's family had been very influential supporters of the medical center, and the ax was swift and powerful. The resident's error was careless and revealed immaturity at a minimum, but there was no malice of thought. Nevertheless, it was a huge mistake that altered his career substantially. The issue was not the conversation—the discussion was relevant and appropriate to have with a colleague, but it should have been held in strict privacy.

Patients have a right to expect complete confidentially whatever their medical concern; however, with information pertaining to cancer privacy becomes an obsession with some. Old stigmas endure, and certain patients want to keep the issue confidential. This is especially important in some high-profile patients in which the reason for privacy is obvious. In other patients, however, the obsession with keeping the cancer private might be based on not wanting family members to worry or simply not wishing to constantly be perceived in the shadow of the illness.

During the period in which I practiced at Georgetown University Medical Center in the nation's capital, I had the opportunity to take care of a number of national leaders, many well known and recognizable. We generally catered to them by not requiring waiting-room delays, instead ushering them into exam rooms upon entry into the office. This was as much for security reasons as it was privacy. In any event, I was seeing a prominent member of the president's cabinet—the secretary of an important department of government. He came through the waiting area with a bodyguard and was quickly brought into an exam room. I examined him, and we made plans for an operation. Then he was ushered out—all within forty-five minutes. That same night, on network news, it was announced that Secretary "So and So" had visited a Georgetown cancer surgeon that day for an unknown reason. The firestorm began about thirty minutes after the news broadcast, and it started with the leadership of the university. The assumption, of course, had been that we had somehow leaked the information. After checking with the clerical people in my office, all of whom adamantly denied violating this inflexible rule, we started studying the list of other patients who had been in the waiting room that day. A producer for the reporting network was on the patient list, and when I called him and asked the question, he readily admitted that the information had come from him. Even though he apologized, he truly felt that he was only doing his job. I was aggravated by this, but accepted his explanation and reported back to the secretary, who, as it turned out, understood the game far better than I, and all was forgiven. The beltway insider understood the fundamental fact that the newsman reporting that information was different from our having leaked it. In the latter circumstance, it would have been an unforgivable violation of patient confidentiality.

When caring for famous people, there can be great pressure on the doctor from outside sources—news media, gossip columnists, and social acquaintances who somehow are aware that the patient is under medical care. Whatever the source, and no matter how relentless the pressure, the patient's privacy must be regarded as sacrosanct. On a number of occasions, my wife and children have been surprised to learn from an outside source that a famous person was under my care, but they always understood why they had not heard it from me.

I did violate that confidence one time, many years ago. I had been asked to go to a country in Central America to examine and care for the president of that country. Because there was some concern of an impending coup, he was unable to come to the medical center where I was an attending surgeon. The potential adventure was too much for me to resist, and I flew there in an unmarked plane dispatched by that country's military. Upon landing, I was whisked off the plane at the end of the runway and taken to the palace, where I examined the president; we made arrangements for surgery to be done that same night. The procedure was done under tight security, with armed guards in the operating room. Fortunately, the problem was easily corrected. Several days later, after making sure my patient was doing well, I left under the same security blanket as before. Back in my home base, I returned to my routine. Two days later a very large man with a crew cut and a dark suit and tie came to my office to ask about my recent visit to that Central American country. He was from the CIA, and he wanted to know what my business with that particular president had been. I stammered and hesitated under the unsmiling stare of a very intimidating guy, and after partially recovering from the revelation that my secret trip had been anything but a secret, I ended up telling him more than I had planned to, and certainly more than I should have. I have always rationalized my breach of that president's confidentiality by telling myself that since this was not a cancer-related problem my transgression was not as serious as it might have been. I wonder how resolute I would have been in circumstances where cancer was the issue, in which confidentiality would be more important. I am embarrassed to admit that, because I was frightened, I did not "practice what I preached." I fully confessed all of this to my patient. Not only did he readily forgive me but he was greatly amused and somehow not surprised that the CIA was so interested in him.

One of the pitfalls that some doctors encounter while caring for cancer-afflicted celebrities—whether they be captains of industry, financiers, athletes, politicians, show-business types, or even Mafia dons—is that they are frequently surrounded by aides and other members of an entourage who feel obligated and empowered to be protective. Additionally, the celebrity is often accustomed to people jumping on command, and the minions can be very demanding in seeking to create an environment of subservience around their boss. A friend of mine spent four years as the U.S. president's personal physician, and his travails in dealing with his patient's subordinates vastly exceeded that of the boss. No physician should participate in the charade conjured up by such a team. Instead, the doctor should uphold the dignity of the profession and at all times do only that which is medically in the best interest of the patient and that which follows the highest of standards. A sense of protectiveness for the patient must be part of a physician's credo and leadership skill set. Surprisingly, most patients recognize the value of such an attitude, just as do high-profile and powerful people, who, with proper handling, can also be some of the nicest and most grateful patients.

Physicians who take care of famous patients must be guarded about compromising care by catering to their whims because of their star power; they usually understand the word "no." Especially in surgery, we scrupulously and compulsively follow certain routines for the simple reason that they are best for achieving the goals of the operation. While the physician can be impressed by someone's accomplishments or fame, showing respect and deference by making allowances for issues of security and privacy, patient care should be standard state of the art, and it should be recommended and administered with the same leadership and take-charge approach that the oncologist routinely uses. Even people of substance and wisdom may unconsciously test the boundaries of control, but in the end, they usually respond with relief and appreciation when a physician takes charge and does not allow patient dominance. With that said, it is important for physicians to be certain of their own motives and ensure that their behavior is not designed merely to prove a point. There are occasions when the patient correctly questions the method recommended, sometimes for reasons of which the physician is unaware. Within the bounds of good medical care, the physician should be flexible, depending on the request. I will speak more about the power and control issues that relate to the physician-patient relationship, but at this point, suffice it to say that special patients should be leery of special treatment by physicians who are star struck.

No matter how elevated or important, most intelligent cancer patients want their cancer physician to demonstrate leadership with a thoughtful and cogent game plan for dealing with their tumor. This is not always an easy status to achieve, especially early in an oncologist's career. I remember very well when I was a young attending surgeon on the faculty in the Texas Medical Center in the mid-1970s being asked to see a patient for a vocal cord cancer. R.C. was the quintessential Texas oilman in appearance and deeds. His name was the stuff of legend in Houston, and his family epitomized the very Texas tradition of supporting local institutions. They had done that through personal action and leadership, as well as with vast amounts of money donated to their beloved and world famous Texas Medical Center. The patient was dominant and charming, commanding attention whenever he walked into a room. His presence was like that of the proverbial 800-pound gorilla, a force impossible to ignore. R.C. had earned his measure of deference over Germany during World War II, and afterward in the tough world of the Texas oil industry. In the language that is uniquely Texan, this was an important person.

On that first visit, I walked into the exam room to find a large man engulfed in a cloud of smoke, as he sat with a large cigar clenched between his teeth. R.C. looked at me, and casually took the cigar out of his mouth, but kept it at a close distance in his hand. The slight smile that developed as I came forward is impossible to describe—neither welcoming nor sardonic, but anticipatory, and when combined with a perfectly elevated eyebrow, betraying real skepticism of this youngster who had just walked into the room. I could almost feel the words that were on his mind—"Your move, sonny. What ya gonna do about it?" I didn't have to be a psychologist to realize that I was in a control struggle of the first magnitude. The struggle continued with a handshake of epic proportions, undoubtedly designed to test my manhood.

"Doctor, it's nice to meet you," he said as he looked deep inside me.

I responded appropriately, while wondering how long it would be before I got my hand back. During that time of subliminal combat, the eye contact was not unfriendly, but was intense. Finally, he asked as he handled the cigar like a thing of interest, "The smoke bother you?"

I didn't take the bait. "No not at all," I said. "Actually I like good cigars."

"Oh . . . well let me send you a box. They're Cubans," he said.

"Thanks, but I'll pass," I said, "I quit smoking some time ago, and having them around would be tempting."

The smile warmed a tad, perhaps as a result of finding commonality with a physician who was also vulnerable to the seduction of nicotine.

I then got my hand back, and that is when I made my move for control of the situation, with some desire to also restore my dignity. "I do want you to put out your cigar, however. Medical Center rules, you know, and besides, it makes it a little hard to examine your throat."

He laughed, extinguished the cigar, and said, "I'm sorry, Doctor. I should have thought of that."

I thought, but of course didn't say, "Sure, I'll bet you hadn't thought of it." In the antismoking climate of today, this story seems almost unimaginable, but this was the mid-1970s, and even though completely inappropriate, his behavior was less unusual at the time, and let's not overlook that he "was who he was," so to speak. As I came to know this really fine man, he never would admit that his smoking in the exam room was an intentional provocation, although he did smile when the story came up.

Happily, R.C. was cured of his cancer and went on to live a number of years afterward, during which he and his family continued their generous support for the Texas Medical Center. To my chagrin, however, I never got him to quit smoking, although he never again lit up in the office. Furthermore, I don't think that he really believed that I had quit smoking; months after his treatment was completed, I received a box of Cuban cigars in the mail—sender unrevealed. Except for cheating on the smoking issue, this man had become a delightful patient and friend, and could not have been more of a gentleman, even if not an ideal patient.

While wanting leadership from their cancer physician, patients don't often engage in the initial tug of war that I just described. Most powerful individuals do, however, want to hear a cogent plan of action, a grasp of subject matter, and decisiveness in their physician. They are comforted if they understand what they are told and, appropriately, annoyed if they do not.

Physician flexibility must be tempered with experience, maturity, and firmness. I remember well a situation faced by a colleague of mine who was an esteemed surgical oncologist at a famous cancer center. He was a leading international authority on the cancer for which he was treating a very successful national politician. The person in question wanted to run for the presidency, but to reveal the need for a cancer operation would obviously have compromised his viability as a candidate. The patient and the patient's minions opted to delay treatment until after the political process, a course that was strongly discouraged by my colleague. The politician was not nominated, and after almost a year of delay, eventually got around to taking care of the cancer. My friend operated, but things had progressed substantially, and the person went on to die from a malignancy that probably would have been cured if treated in a timely fashion. My colleague had cared for many important people, and although very fond of this particular patient, was thoroughly unimpressed by his star status. He had been adamant in his advice to operate earlier, but unfortunately the twin demons of vanity and ambition won over judgment, and good medical advice was ignored.

· 14 ·

Essentials of Communication Skills: Listening, Hearing, Reading Body Language

$\mathcal{O}$f all of the attributes of the effective oncologist, being a good listener is one of the most important. For some time, I have been impressed how patients often instinctively have a sense of their own body, and on many occasions feel something is wrong well before telltale symptoms or signs cause concern for their physician. While studying physical diagnosis, medical students are frequently admonished to "listen to what your patient is saying; they will often give you valuable information that you aren't even seeking." So when a patient says that "something is wrong," the wise doctor will take heed.

In these circumstances, the admonition is generally meant to apply to diagnostic problems; however, the statement also applies to the routines of medical practice. Such is the case when a patient is telling you what has transpired with other physicians or other treatments. Not infrequently, patients come from a referring doctor confused and ill informed about their tumor, and its potential treatment. At first glance, one is tempted to fault the referring doctor, but in truth, the explanation for this state is usually complicated. First, some doctors are simply not good at teaching or explaining, and even when time permits, the communication is ineffective. Second, misunderstandings, misperceptions, and superstitions often result from fear of the most dreaded word in language—*cancer*, or as it is colloquially known, the "Big C."[1]

So even when the referring doctor does a good job of explaining, not surprisingly, patients often do not understand or do not remember. And because they are embarrassed or too considerate of the doctor's hectic schedule, they do not ask for further explanation. So sometimes these patients leave the primary physician with a referral slip in hand but confused and with marginal knowledge.

Between this visit and the time of the consultation with the cancer specialist, in addition to forgetting more of the factual information, they and their families often cloud an already emotional situation by talking to other patients or friends of patients who are quick to give unsolicited advice. Hearsay information is often inaccurate and overly dramatized, and for many reasons, the recipient forgets to factor in the commonsense axiom that what applies to one patient does not necessarily apply to another. In an attempt to be helpful, friends, relatives, and other self-appointed advisors can be counterproductive in their efforts and, while well-meaning, can do real harm to the patient's state of mind during the journey between diagnosis and treatment completion. Even though most cancer patients intuitively know that it's unwise to listen to nonmedical advisors, especially the self-appointed ones, in the real world of cancer hysteria, they often do just that. Human nature and unchecked verbosity have probably overridden common sense and caution for as long as people have interacted. The power of emotions to trump logic is a veritable force of nature, and one of the first jobs of the treating physician is to overcome much of what has developed during the interval between the referral and the visit to the cancer physician. Because misconceptions and partial truths that result from faulty communications are sometimes hard to overcome, this issue is important at this particular point of the book, which is devoted to communication skills.

That a patient is susceptible to the advice and influence of another layperson often means that the referring physician or even the treating physician has not really connected and communicated. It is important not to confuse this with wrongdoing on the physician's part; instead, it usually reflects a lack of recognition by the physician that the patient was unclear about what was explained. Having said this, it should be noted that even though unintentional, the failure to read the patient's countenance and body language usually represents a deficiency in the physician's communication skills. It's essential to recognize whether you have gotten through to a patient, and it shouldn't be necessary to hold a quiz after the conversation. I say that somewhat in jest, but occasionally I do in fact ask several basic questions in order to judge if the patient has understood what was explained. This practice is often unreliable, however, and can be embarrassing for the patient; therefore, this quizzing method must only be employed with great conversational finesse.

Gaining the Patient's Confidence

$\mathcal{T}$he referring doctor's recommendation of a particular cancer specialist should involve the thoughtful choice of a person with both the skill set for the job as well as the personality to stimulate and sustain a meaningful physician-patient relationship through interactive and thoughtful communication skills. Actually, the groundwork for that future relationship starts in the office of the referring doctor. More than just handing the patient a piece of paper with a name on it, some profile information on the specialist and his or her attributes ought to be given. It is especially reassuring when referring doctors say something to the effect that they would not hesitate to send a member of their own family to this particular cancer specialist. Additionally, referrers should warn about the hazards of unsolicited and unsophisticated advice during the time before the visit to the cancer specialist. Finally, referring doctors should advise patients about the potential presence of an audience—that is, residents, medical students, nurses, and others—often present in the medical center environment, especially when in a university hospital. All of this attention can be especially daunting for cancer patients and their loved ones. It can be an intimidating event for a frightened and vulnerable patient when a highly touted oncologist—surgical, radiation, or medical—walks into a room with an aura of professorial confidence among doting residents and students. Finally, the referring doctor should encourage the patient and family to advocate for themselves but at the same time to do their share to nurture the relationship with the oncologist to whom they are referred. The bond that hopefully develops is often tested as the very scary journey of cancer diagnosis and treatment is made.

It should be clear by this point that the referring doctor has a responsibility to solicit and listen to patient feedback on the oncologists to whom patients were sent previously. When I refer a patient to another doctor, or when I bring in other members of the cancer team, I always at some point ask the patient about the other physician. By that time, I have been brought up to speed on the progress of what has been done, but the query to which I refer relates to the patient's perception of that person. I do not seek a grade but only an instinctive human response. Before I incorporate another physician into the team, I always ask myself if I would entrust a member of my own family to that particular person. Is the personality match good? Is the considered physician verbal enough for this patient? Perhaps one particular patient needs a more effective explainer—one not prone to abruptness or impatience. Above all, even though arrogance is never an admirable trait, it is especially offensive in someone in whom so much power is entrusted, and unless there is a compelling reason to overlook this aggravating trait, I choose someone else.

Recently, my wife and I had dinner with a couple with whom we had little acquaintance; in fact, prior to the evening in question, we had only exchanged greetings as we passed each other in the neighborhood. That evening, however, as our respective backgrounds entered the conversation, I mentioned that I had been at a certain institution during a certain time in my life. Immediately, the conversation turned to the sad death of their only son, who had been treated at that institution almost thirty years before. He had died of a high-grade sarcoma of the lower spine and pelvic bone. It had apparently been only partially responsive to the usual chemo-radiation therapy protocol, and the operation that ensued had led to substantial weakness of both legs. Worse, the margins of resection were not clear of the tumor, and a second operation was recommended that would have left him with a permanent colostomy, impotence, urinary incontinence, and finally half a pelvis and one leg. He was in his mid-twenties at the time, and had not been married. After much soul searching, the young man declined the surgery, despite the aggravation of and extreme pressure from the medical oncologist to "go for it." Instead, the patient decided to seek alternative measures, which consisted of a macrobiotic diet. Not surprisingly, this failed, and he died at home several months later.

As my wife and I listened to these very reasonable and educated parents, their bitterness was impossible to ignore. I remained silent, despite the fact that I knew the medical team well, and, in fact, the lead oncologist was internationally known for his management of this particular tumor. My reason for not contributing was twofold: They didn't invite my comments; and second, despite the passage of thirty years since the death of this young man, the couple's verbal catharsis seemed appropriate and perhaps was therapeutic. Several days later I received a large envelope in my mailbox that contained the daily journal the young man had kept during the whole terrible sequence of events.

Additionally, there was a copy of a well-known newspaper that had featured an article based on his daily log. A friend of his who worked as a journalist had wanted to share this sad story with the readership. Also included in my mailbox was a copy of a rebuttal letter written to the newspaper's chief editor by the lead oncologist, who had been pushing so hard for the surgery. The letter reflected a total lack of sensitivity to the terrible emotional ordeal that his proposed operation created for this young man. The thrust of the doctor's rebuttal letter was that it was irresponsible for the newspaper to publish such an article because it would compromise the willingness of future patients to undergo similar life-saving surgery.

After studying all of this, I contacted my neighbor and asked him why he still harbored such bitterness—obviously sadness over the loss of a child is permanent, but I wanted to better understand the resentment. Even though I strongly suspected the reason before he explained, I wanted to hear it from him in an unfettered fashion.

"First and foremost," he said, "the arrogance of the lead oncologist was amazing, and his total lack of sensitivity to the situation was then and will always remain unforgivable." He added that the family felt excluded from the information, no one counseled them, and in general they were able to get information only under duress and through the patient. He admitted to the high quality of the care, but was infuriated by how they were all handled. I said to him that he had a right to be angry and that based on my reading of his son's journal and my knowledge of their oncologist (I had shared care of a number of patients with him) I would feel the same way. Essentially, I apologized to him on behalf of a very arrogant physician and a fine institution.

Accuracy of interpretation after the fact is perhaps subject to exaggeration, but in this case, I think not. Hopefully, in the ensuing years, we have gotten better at "these psychological things." When one considers this situation, we couldn't have been much worse. What is important here is the perception of the family. The exclusion from the process in an event that probably ranks with the most intense in the human experience, and the fact that this father has kept this file at his fingertips for all these years indicates only in small measure the emotional ferocity of his feelings.

· *16* ·

The Cancer Specialist as a Teacher of the Patient and Family: The Lead-Up to Treatment

*T*he referral of a cancer patient to the appropriate specialist is a critical first step in a chain of events, because it usually is the entry point to a particular cancer team. So indirectly, at least, the selection of the team is influenced by the thoughtful family doctor's choice of lead cancer specialist. Obviously, the referral is a step undertaken only after having done one's homework. Once assigned, the patient's initial task is to remain open and trusting of the chosen team, adhering to the game plan that is developed and recommended. Further consultation and second opinions are useful and should be encouraged, but at the end of the day, ruminations must cease and the patient and family have to get on board with the people and the chosen strategy.

Once the process starts, things tend to occur automatically and sequentially, and while not impossible, it is a huge endeavor and frequently a compromise of standards, to change teams in mid-stream. If confidence in the cancer team is not present at the outset, therefore, the situation is fundamentally flawed, and must be rethought. I will go even further by saying that patients that do not have absolute trust in their oncologist—whether surgical, radiation, or medical—should make other arrangements before the treatment starts. Conversely, if a physician senses a lack of trust in the patient or the family, he or she should promptly confront the situation and resolution should be sought. If this is not possible, the patient should find alternate medical care. Importantly, the mere presence of the doubts is significant and must be promptly resolved, regardless of the reasons for them. Even though this crossroad in the physician-patient relationship is potentially wounding to some of those involved, bold confrontation is needed because without resolution, the seed is sowed for discontent and negative behavior. As I reflect on these matters, I am reminded of the words of George Eliot, "What loneliness is more lonely then distrust."[1] Much like jealousy, distrust is erosive and wastes emotional energy. It should be noted that once the responsibility for a patient's care has been accepted, the physician does not have the legal or ethical privilege of merely refusing to continue care; instead, alternative arrangements must be made if severance of the relationship is desired.

The whole trust issue is especially important in strong individuals who are accustomed to controlling their life and, not infrequently, the lives of the people around them. Clearly, control and trust are inextricably linked; it would be daunting for anyone to think of putting his or her life into the hands of a virtual stranger, no matter how decorated their curriculum vitae. Ideally this high level of mutual commitment grows after the patient and cancer specialist begin to interact, but the groundwork should begin long before with the credibility and integrity of the referring doctor, on whom the patient depends.

Earlier, I mentioned that patients who are referred to an oncologist not infrequently are confused and ill informed, and I further suggested that the fault was generally not entirely that of the referring doctor but related to a complex array of issues. Nevertheless, we must separate fault from responsibility. Whatever the cause of the breakdown is, patient comprehension should ultimately be the responsibility of the doctor, not the patient. Why the physician should shoulder that degree of responsibility for comprehension has to do with the physiology of a frightened person. Let me explain.

For some time, I have been impressed how cancer patients, no matter how intelligent, retain only a portion of what they initially are told. With repetition, the retention percentage goes up in a linear way, but initially that portion is surprisingly small. The memory is fickle, and despite the tenacity of unpleasant facts, the brain seems to serve as an effective filtration system by eliminating the bad in favor of the good. The scientific proof may be inadequate to defend this, but most observant physicians have witnessed such a phenomenon. Many doctors try to counteract this tendency by writing explanatory letters to patients summarizing and reinforcing what was discussed. Unfortunately, however, some physicians don't stress patient comprehension, the result being patient ignorance and confusion, both of which can complicate matters on numerous levels and thwart the development of the physician-patient relationship. If complications or even failure of the treatment strategy occur, the patient who is confused or uninformed is more likely to feel betrayed and angry.

Obviously, some patients are more sophisticated and more intelligent than others, and the explanations must be tailored to the appropriate level. The ability to phrase language appropriately and to judge receptivity by observing the countenance of a patient are essential to a cancer physician's communicative skills. People of limited intelligence can be overwhelmed with even a straightforward topic that has been presented with a rhetorical flourish—wordy in scientific phraseology and seemingly designed to impress, rather than explain. I have heard physicians give an overview of the disease in great detail and a long-term strategy that can involve multiple cancer teams—surgical oncologist, radiation oncologists, medical oncologists, psycho-oncologists, dentists, nurses, nutritionists, social workers—all in one verbal dose delivered within the course of several minutes and immediately after telling a patient that he has cancer. This is unacceptable. Confirmation of the cancer diagnosis is, in itself, extraordinary. When combined with a complex game plan it's little wonder that some patients and families are overwhelmed. However achieved, the complexities of the conversation must be distilled, transmitted, and received in a comprehensible way. Again, I emphasize the premise that it is the responsibility of the physician to insure that this happens.

I remember very well sitting with my wife about ten years ago in the office of a New York City dermatologist who outlined the strategy for doing on her what is called Mohs Surgery for an aggressive facial skin cancer. The doctor sat reciting scripted information about tumor margins, processing, scar potential, other possible complications, and more—all delivered in rapid, memorized fashion, with little eye contact, and in such a way that even I, as a cancer surgeon, had to strain to understand. It was clear to my very intelligent wife that it would be easier to pretend comprehension and then have me explain it on the way home. Needless to say, the whole process annoyed her. Had I not been available to translate the doctor's obligatory speech, she would have resentfully felt a need to advocate for herself and ask numerous questions. In the final analysis, an important level of confidence in the plan or the team would not have existed. There had been no familiarity, no warmth, no "laying on of the hands," and no sense of protectiveness on the part of the doctor. And as a result, a relationship that would have carried my wife through problems was never established. Fortunately, the procedure was uneventful and the outcome was good, but if that had not been the case, the stage was set for a very unhappy patient. I'm still convinced that this particular surgeon didn't have the slightest clue that the climate was less than ideal. After all was said and done, I was tempted to bring all of this up, but realizing the usual futility of trying to educate a middle-aged person on basic human communication, I decided against it.

There is a difference between the physician who does not understand how to communicate and the one who fails to communicate because of a lack of commitment to patient autonomy or unconcern about the psychological impact that can result from the information. Both situations are blatantly unacceptable in the medical climate of today. Before current standards were adopted, patients were told only what their doctor felt they should know. In part, this reflected an arrogance that automatically assumed the patient was incapable of understanding nuance. I don't believe that those doctors were any less humane or compassionate—they were then, as we are now, mostly generous, unselfish, and dedicated to the improvement of the human condition. Instead, I would like to think that their behavior reflected "the times," in which patients demanded little and doctors offered less in the way of explanation. Their conclusions, recommendations, and proclamations were virtually sacrosanct—not to be questioned. In that bygone era, patients had few rights, and only the most inquisitive and demanding patients challenged the explanations of their physician.

That sort of behavior was not limited to the medical profession, however. The same was true for all authority figures—legal, educational, and others. Dogma from the elite was the norm, and the Patient's Bill of Rights that is posted in all medical facilities today was then unthinkable. The Informed Consent forms of today were equally nonexistent, and in general, when doctors did explain, they were poorly understood because a priority was not placed on patient comprehension.

Communicative skills are but a part of general "people skills," many of which are learned during one's upbringing. Teaching young doctors the art of communication is no small task, even when the basic familial foundation is in place. In many success stories throughout all walks of life—medical and otherwise—good communication skills are a key ingredient of the abilities of the successful individual. The reader is reminded that communication consists of two components—that given and that received. So, informing the patient and the family is not necessarily the same as communicating with them. No matter how loquacious the physician, if he or she has not been understood, the goal has not been achieved. A monologue occurs when one-person talks, dialogue when two verbally interact—communication can result from either, but there must be mutual understanding.

Comprehension early on is critical in cancer patients, since the stakes are usually higher and there are often treatment options. Importantly, the life of the cancer patient—even after being cured—is never quite the same. As early as medical school, I felt that an informed patient was an asset to the care that one administers. My father had great communication skills, and I either inherited that or learned by his example. I suspect both factors have gone into my ability to transmit an understandable message to patients. I was, therefore, fortunate to start out with a base of explanatory ease, and I have continued to work on those skills. As I advanced in my career, gaining self-confidence along the way, I became a more effective communicator.

Having already established that I believe the ultimate measurement of effective communication is a patient's comprehension, I am quick to add that actually getting to that state is another matter. As an academic, I have spent my life attempting to teach—not pontificate without concern for comprehension—but teach in a manner that leads to understanding. Whether with young doctors or patients, the gold standard ought to be clarity. It's actually easier to teach young physicians than patients because the teacher generally doesn't escape until the matter is clear. Patients are less inclined to self-advocacy; therein is the reason for being perceptive to a patient's countenance and body language.

Even when teaching comes easily and naturally, the cancer physician should continue to work at becoming better and more effective with patients and their families. For them to really understand is an accomplishment that cannot be overrated and that adds immeasurably to the overall tolerability of the cancer experience. Additionally, the physician can control other factors that help establish a physician-patient connection; however, such refinements only result from thoughtful study of the endeavor and an ongoing honing of one's techniques. Being attentive to the patient's response to various communication techniques is critical to a physician learning what works best.

One's powers of observation and one's ability to listen are fundamental to the process. My suggestion to young doctors is to observe their various mentors—take from them what seems uniquely effective. Never be condescending about learning from everyone, no matter how humble the person's relative station in the medical system. Many physicians in small-town America, for example, have considerable skill and common sense regarding the art of medicine. All through the mentorship experience, the young doctor should add whatever personal methods suit his or her individual style. Throughout the years, doctors will also learn what not to do by watching the interpersonal ineptness of some of their colleagues. Eventually, an eclectic style of practicing and communicating is developed. With this method of mentoring the American system of medical education has the advantage over the traditional European method, in which one professor is the filter of most information, and the eclectic style is discouraged.

Aside from those methods over which a physician has control, good fundamental chemistry with a patient helps greatly—and when it is present, patients are more willing to interact in dialogue and ask questions that lead to comprehension. As in all walks of life, people who like each other have an easier time with such things. With that said, it is important to note that familiarity does not necessarily lead to good personal chemistry; that is to say, being a "good ol' boy" is not what patients seek in their cancer physician. A lack of arrogance, an honest directness, an ability to listen, a respect for the patient—no matter their station in life—and other intangibles constitute a better formula for likeability. At the opposite end of the spectrum are aloofness and formality, both of which are as unappealing to patients as is the "good ol' boy" persona. Somewhere between rigid formality and a first-name basis seems to be the appropriate place for a cancer physician and a patient to interact—at least in the beginning of the relationship.

I have heard physicians walk into an exam room or up to the patient's bedside and introduce themselves with something parallel to "Hello Alice, I'm Doctor So-and-So." This is especially disrespectful to an older patient, who should always be treated with the deference accorded to one's elders. I remember a friend of mine telling me of an encounter when he thoughtlessly approached an elderly woman with a first-name greeting, and much to his embarrassment, not only were his manners corrected, but he was asked to leave the room. Not only had she not invited his visit, but he introduced himself by his title, while addressing her by her first name. In today's world of political correctness, people are usually taught to use the appropriate language; however, the elderly sometimes are excluded from that protection. Because of my old-fashioned naiveté, I prefer to think that good manners have been around longer than political correctness; however, whichever is the motivating force, the result of addressing people respectfully seems to yield a favorable response more often than not.

Some patients, regardless of age, will open the conversation with a greeting that uses the doctor's first name. I have always wondered how anyone could think this appropriate, but it does happen occasionally. I seek to offset any tendency on the part of patients to go there by introducing myself as Doctor Sessions, and addressing the patient as Mr., Ms., or Mrs.—whichever is appropriate. If a patient ignores these rules of etiquette and continues to call me by my first name, I usually ignore it the first time or two, all the while continuing to address them in the formal way. The message is usually clearly received, and I have never known a patient to continue on the first-name basis under those circumstances. However, if this lack of patient appropriateness were to continue, the situation should be rectified with polite but direct talk.

I go into these things because, even though they are relevant to all early encounters with patients, they are especially important in matters pertaining to cancer. The point was made in an early section of this book that cancer-related medical care is a sober endeavor that deals with serious issues and achieving the proper interaction mandates the establishment of the alpha position of authority for the physician. As things move along, and after the operational systems and emotional bonds have developed, it is often appropriate and acceptable if a less formal attitude is adopted. In my experience, just when and under which circumstances informality is appropriate usually becomes obvious. I made the point earlier that familiarity does not necessarily lead to good interpersonal chemistry; the same is true of informality. Call me old fashioned, but I believe that patients want to defer to their physicians.

Another physician-controlled enhancement to communication with a cancer patient is a state of relaxation that allows the patient not to feel rushed. A patient wants to feel that they have a physician's full attention, without the sense that they are trying to get out the door. If a patient doesn't get that feeling, a comfort zone is unachievable and they feel the need to hurriedly make important points. A great technique for accomplishing this state of relaxation is for the physician to sit down—in an exam room setting on a nearby chair, or if in the hospital, on a chair or even on the edge of the patient's bed. Even if for a very short time, doing so indicates a relaxed focus on what the patient is telling you. Obviously, the conversation has to be governed by the physician, because some patients have difficulty staying on track. With some effort, however, this is usually easy to accomplish.

An aura of physician self-confidence is also important to effective communication. Importantly, this should be derived from strength of personality and the self-assurance that allows patients to ask penetrating questions and seek real answers. This sense of self is totally different from cockiness or arrogance, neither of which should have a home in dealing with cancer patients and their families. Achieving this state of mind becomes easier for the physician with age and experience, and a record of achievement. However, such a state is not limited to older physicians. Many young and freshly trained oncologists have that intangible quality that is immediately obvious to colleagues and patients alike, and patients are undeniably comforted by its presence.

The Physician as an Educator after Treatment: Using the Cancer as a Tool

In the course of management of a cancer, an important part of the oncologist's responsibility is to educate and to direct both the patient and the family to information sources. It should always be remembered that the family—children, grandchildren, and others—even if not present during the educational process, indirectly get the message about cancer prevention, early diagnosis, and a generally optimistic overview of our capabilities in the war against this disease.

Allow me to use a hypothetical scenario that I have actually orchestrated many times during my career to illustrate a teaching exercise. As almost everyone on the planet knows smoking is bad for you, and is especially problematic in the upper aero-digestive tract, where it is a carcinogen. Tobacco use—smokeless or smoking, whether by chewing, cigar, pipe, and cigarettes—whether filtered or unfiltered—is directly related to the development of a very high percentage of the cancers of the upper aero-digestive tract and lung. There are exceptions in which patients afflicted with certain carcinomas of the aero-digestive area have not used tobacco products, and for them we look to genetic factors and certain types of viral infections. However, in tobacco users—especially smokers—the cause-and-effect relationship is clear and irrefutable. Since my career as a head and neck cancer surgeon has been dominated by the management of tobacco-related cancers, I have spent a staggering amount of time in the aggregate talking about this issue to patients, and because of the pulpit provided by my academic positions, I have also expounded over television, in congressional testimony, and in other venues. While those public responsibilities are a serious part of the responsibility of the academic leadership of medicine, this book is more about physician–cancer patient matters, and the experiences in educating patients and families is the point of this section. The "stop smoking discussion" is essential early in the course of the relationship between cancer patient and physician. First and foremost, the oncologist must not equivocate in this matter; call a fact a fact—the proof is there. No one, not even those associated with the tobacco industry, denies it. I frequently will even say to patients that it is important that their children or grandchildren know what got you to this point so they won't deceive themselves into thinking that smoking is not dangerous. "Something positive may as well come out of your smoking," I tell patients, unapologetically playing on their sense of guilt and responsibility to their family. At the same time, this technique incorporates family members who in addition to passing on the information to others will hopefully also support the patient's determination to quit the habit. Children, especially daughters, can be ferocious watchdogs when it comes to keeping a parent on the straight and narrow.

I am dogmatic and graphic with these patients, and tend to lay it on with a bit of flourish. Even if the patient has only a premalignant lesion in the upper aero-digestive tract, I will lean hard, flexing "prediction muscles" by saying to them, "if you continue to smoke, it's not a matter of if, but when you will have a cancer." In truth, while resulting cancer is not a certainty, it is highly likely. If the cancer is already present, and we are about to launch treatment, I am even more dogmatic: "Your chances of both treatment success and cure are a lot less if you continue to smoke." Then I explain my reasoning: First, if they are to have surgery, compromise in the circulation caused by nicotine-induced spasm of the blood vessels makes the wound less likely to heal. Additionally, the overall surgical complication rate increases substantially. This applies to all surgery, and all cancer operations, whether the smoke has been the cause of the cancer or not. Second, if the patient is to get radiation, either before or after the surgery, or even if there is to be only radiation, the effectiveness of the radiation depends in part on the proper oxygenation of tissue. It follows that since blood vessels deliver oxygen to all body tissue, and since smoking causes spasm and constriction of the small vessels, there is a resulting decrease of the blood, and therefore, in the tissue's oxygen supply. "The term for this is tissue hypoxia, but that's doctor talk," I tell them, "and I want you to realize that this idea is not complicated. The bottom line is that you have less chance for cure and less chance for healing." The grand finale of my pitch is to say, "There's a good chance that we can cure this cancer, but if you continue or start smoking again, your chance of developing another cancer—not the same one, but a different second cancer in the same general area—is very high, maybe 70 percent or so." I add, "If you get another one, we generally don't have as many options for treatment the next time around. For example, we often are not able to use radiation in the same area again, and whatever surgery is required at the time is likely to be fairly radical."

After this "tough love" approach, I put things on a personal level. I understand just how hard it is to quit this terrible habit. I know from personal experience, and many years after stopping, I still periodically have the urge to smoke. I use this when making my pitch to get people to stop, saying that I was a heavy smoker for years, and I don't minimize the difficulties they face. Actually, I have always felt that people who have never been addicted to nicotine find it hard to comprehend these difficulties. Without question, the cancer is the best motivator, but even with this, it's amazing how many people would return to the dark side if the medical team were not actively involved with commonsense education and encouragement, constantly reminding them and staying with them when they slip off the wagon. Despite our best efforts, some nonetheless succumb to the habit and go back to smoking.

Throughout all of this, there exists the underlying theme of physicians being the protectors—paternalistic, if you wish—who view etiologic and sociologic issues as being within their purview, and who accept as part of the mission the continued involvement with the psyche of the patient. I view this concept as basic responsibility. Who better to influence the patient than the person who has treated their cancer?

The opportunity for the education of the younger generation often comes as a result of the cancer experience of a parent or other relative. Showing the destructiveness of tobacco is the most obvious of these educational tools, but this same general approach can be used with information about breast cancer and estrogens, and explaining preventative measures such as mammography, uterine cytology (pap smear), colonoscopy, prostate screening, skin protection, human papillomavirus vaccine, and others. Cancer physicians must take the lead along with other segments of the profession in educating the next generation, and the experience of family members surviving cancer is the most effective tool at their disposal.

· 18 ·

The Journey from the Referring Doctor to the Oncologist: Uncertainty, Anxiety, and Hope along the Way

Cancer patients are generally referred to oncologists from other physicians— primary care, gynecologists, endocrinologists, pulmonologists, gastroenterologists, otolaryngologists, and others. Not uncommonly, at the time of their initial visit with the surgeon or one of the other oncologists, the patient is unclear as to whether they have a malignancy. Many of them had been told, but they did not hear what they did not want to hear. This is a good example of what I meant earlier when I referred to the brain as a filtration system for frightening information.

In situations in which there is suspicion but no proof of cancer, the referring doctor may have told them, "You have a problem," or "You have a tumor," or "You have a growth," but often even that is unclear in their mind. Regarding this type of phraseology, many doctors seek to avoid delivering bad news, so it's entirely correct for them to skirt around the cancer or malignancy words until proof is actually established. In most patients, the use of the slightly evasive terms such as "a problem," "a tumor," or "a growth" is enough, unless the next step of arranging for an oncologist is delayed. However, patients will sometimes push the referring physician to speculate, and this tricky conversation should be avoided. If the patient asks directly, "Could it be malignant?" the physician should be honest with a simple yes—after all, why else would the patient be referred to a cancer specialist. Even though the physician's concern is enough to raise the patient's anxiety level, many referrers wisely choose not to speculate on likelihood or other specifics.

One is tempted to comfort the patient, but on many occasions, such an attempt will introduce unrealistic expectations. In certain circumstances, it is appropriate for a referring physician to offer general data that is favorable and that would give a patient cause for hope. For instance, approximately 80 percent of "incidentally" discovered breast masses in women turn out to be nonmalignant. Similar optimism is possible in a patient with a parotid gland tumor, in which about 75 percent are benign. Quoting such generic data when sending the patient for a diagnostic procedure is different from specifically making predictions about that particular patient's mass. In the case of a potentially ominous tumor—a pancreas tumor for instance—no real value is gained by speculating on the dismal statistics associated with this group of malignancies. In many cancers, the probability of cure is directly stage-related, and in the process of quoting overall numbers, the bad is included with the good. Better the patient be properly worked up and staged and the prognosis developed based on the specific tumor burden.

Once the cancer word is mentioned, fear takes hold and the patient can become relentless in asking questions that the referring physician is really unable to answer. Many patients will not ask for speculation or predictions out of fear of hearing dreaded news; others will. In an effort to avoid this trap, referring physicians are often intentionally vague. This is not an incorrect or unethical technique; on the contrary it gives the oncologist latitude to develop the discussion in a more positive and factually based manner.

The suspicion of cancer having been raised, it is essential that prompt arrangements be made for seeing the oncologist. Except for extraordinary circumstances, it is unacceptable for there to be more than a one-week delay in seeing the one person who is able to answer the question on everyone's mind. The same can be said for delays in obtaining a biopsy and, once done, waiting for the result. This can be a period of emotional agony, and I have been appalled when I have heard of delays of eight to ten days that some patients are asked to endure. Happily, this occurs infrequently. For those readers unfamiliar with the technologic capabilities of modern diagnostic laboratories, the turnover time for a cytology or pathology decision is one to two days, unless special staining techniques are required. In some other circumstances in which diagnostic uncertainty exists, consultation of other cytologists or pathologists more than justifies delay, some of which can be extensive. Most of the time, however, the period needed for diagnostic completion is short, and it is insensitive to drag this out merely for system convenience or a fixed schedule.

In most situations, lumps and bumps—that is, breast masses, swollen lymph nodes, skin lesions, some lung lesions, kidney and liver masses, and others—can be analyzed by needle aspiration and cytology, the arrangements for, and results of which, can be quickly concluded. Even when a more extensive biopsy is indicated, the initial fine needle aspiration can often provide a preliminary diagnosis of malignant or benign. When surgical biopsy is required, some delay is to be expected; however, an effort should be made to prioritize the process. Obviously, these are arbitrary time parameters, and depending on the situation, both the wait for consultation and the wait for the report can be less or more. In general, however, whenever possible, the sooner *the question* is answered the better for the patient. We should always be mindful of the emotional agony of the unknown and uncertainty during that period in limbo.[1] The reader should be clear: I am not advocating time acceleration because of concern for tumor growth—rarely is there a hurry to start treatment. Rather, efficiency and the perception of motion are valuable as being comforting and reassuring to a frightened patient who is anxious to get on with a possible cure.

Thoughtless and insensitive delays are entirely different from the normal time lapse that almost always follows definitive diagnosis—that period in which planning and arrangements are being developed by an oncology team. By the end of this period, the patient has a plan of action, and things are moving forward. Importantly, the patient is occupied with a variety of consultations with the other members of the team, such as radiation and medical oncologists, nurse educators, nutritionists, dentists, psycho-oncologists, social workers, and others. In the cancer management world of today, the sine qua non of excellence is multidisciplinary care; extraordinary arrangements and preparations; treatment decisions and planning in multidisciplinary tumor boards; and an overall seamless interaction of patient, family, and cancer team.

While it is appropriate for the referring doctor to avoid an unpleasant cancer conversation, such is never the case for the oncologist to whom the patient has been referred. Earlier, I described my wife's unhappy experience with the Mohs dermatologist who was the poster child for insensitivity in relaying unpleasant information. Unfortunately, that occurrence is not rare, and it reflects the utter lack of appreciation and concern some physicians display for how to best communicate with a cancer patient. Much as when a teacher tries to judge the effectiveness of what has just been explained, the oncologist must be able to recognize a blank expression that indicates a failure to understand.

With most of my patients, after I have gone over the game plan for disease and treatment strategy, I pose a direct question, "Do you understand what I've told you? If not, I'll be happy to go over it again." It's important for a cancer specialist to realize that some patients are embarrassed by a lack of comprehension, and will try to get past the moment by saying that they do understand when they really don't. For this reason, I often add something like, "It's common for patients to have a lot of questions, and you shouldn't be embarrassed to be a little confused. I realize this is all new information, and maybe I haven't done a good job explaining it." Patients are reassured when a physician demonstrates humility and fallibility. This also serves to make the point that the physician is assuming the responsibility for the comprehension part of communication. At this point, some patients will emphatically say that they really do understand. However, even these patients usually appreciate the extra effort made by the physician.

By this stage, the individual should have a rudimentary grasp of the disease and the game plan for dealing with it. If less comprehension than this is detected, the process should be repeated. No matter how challenging, educating the patient is a wise investment of physician time and often helps to sooth anxiety. The cancer physician must always remember their role as the educator.

Regarding patient education, one should keep in mind that explanations should be adapted to the patient's background and ability to comprehend, and the jargon the physician uses can vary according to the particular individual. The ability to judge the method of discussion is but another of those communication skills that should be in play at all times, and the effectiveness of the explanation must be judged on an individual basis, that is, what works for one patient does not necessarily get through to another.

When possible, the oncologist should map out the planned evaluation leading up to a final decision for a treatment strategy. Most of the time, a tumor board discussion is included in this planning, as are visits to other oncologists if multimodality treatment is a possibility. The patient is then turned over to the staff for appropriate arrangements, and throughout all of this, there should be constant activity. The actions of a sophisticated cancer management team are not limited to the administration of a treatment—radiation, surgery, or chemical—but include planning that is detailed and predictive, driven by the organizational skills of a type of concierge. Such an arranger and implementer can be a nurse or a physician's assistant, both being integral parts of most contemporary cancer teams. Essentially, once a treatment strategy is decided and outlined, the team should be able to tell the patient what will be happening on any specific date and what to expect each step of the way. It is the hallmark of amateurism for the treatment to quickly start without the proper preparation. For example, "We'll try this, and if it doesn't work, we'll worry about alternatives then." Essentially having a game plan from start to finish is ideal.

On the other hand, the sophisticated cancer team should know how to scramble, because on occasion, unforeseen turns occur and it becomes important to be able to alter a carefully laid out strategy. Hopefully, the need to scramble is infrequent, and once a treatment strategy is begun, a major effort is made to see it through on schedule and to completion.

Pushing through a prolonged treatment strategy is not simply about scheduling or organizational convenience, but instead relates to more effective treatment. This is especially important in patients in whom multimodality therapy is being utilized—radiation after surgery, chemotherapy together with radiation, and surgery after radiation are but a few examples in which timing and sequencing are important. Not infrequently, patients experience extraordinary difficulty during radiation, but because the tempo of treatment administration is largely dictated by the physics of nuclear activity and cell cycle concepts, interruption of the plan can be a serious compromise. Stopping therapy because the patient is experiencing difficulty secondary to therapy or has schedule conflicts should be avoided whenever possible. In the treatment of certain head and neck malignancies, and also with certain thoracic tumors, for instance, the side effects of radiation and/or chemotherapy can cause extreme discomfort in swallowing, and whether to press through this misery or to let the patient rest is an important decision. With proper planning, anticipation of such problems often involves the placement of a gastrostomy tube prior to the start of the therapy, circumventing the need to swallow food by a portal for nutrition. Early patient understanding of these possibilities is important because when patients understand the plan, they will try harder to persevere.

Above all, the modern cancer team must remain committed to proven concepts and methods, and the doctor's educational role with the patient and family includes explaining standard methods of management. Pertinent data should be part of the tutorial as long as it is within the capacity of the patient and family to comprehend. In my mind, giving patients choices that are accompanied by data and letting them choose should be preceded by doctors stating what they would recommend to their own family. In doing this, doctors support patients' autonomy and make their decision easier. In my own sphere of interest—the head and neck malignancies—and certain urologic malignancies, such as the prostate gland, there are opportunities for well-informed patients to have real input into their care. Many cancers of these two areas are treated with equal effectiveness by either surgery or radiation therapy. With the exception of certain lymphoid-related malignancies, chemotherapy is not used in a curative manner, but only as an adjunct to surgery or radiation.

In today's cancer centers, tumor board discussions include give and take between the different disciplines, and generally the conclusion of the discussion is characterized by a consensus recommendation for the treating doctor to take back to the patient. With this approach, patients can know specifically what their physician recommends and the consensus of a group as well. If there is a choice in therapies, for example surgery versus radiation therapy, it ought to be presented to the patient with the pros and cons of each being outlined. Most of the time, the patient will express a preference but in the end will usually defer to the opinion of the doctor.

We should always be mindful that in cancer patients, these issues relating to communication and comprehension take on more importance than in noncancer patients. What I call *the cancer experience*—the suspicion, the confirmation, the workup, the treatment, and the follow-up—is a continuum, a journey, if you will, that involves a sustained commitment by a number of individuals.

The family's comprehension should also be considered whenever possible, because as treatment unfolds, their support is often vital; therefore, family members should be included in the planning and explanatory sessions and should be invited to ask questions. This is especially important in certain situations and cultures in which the family unit is particularly cohesive. For example, older couples often have a state of codependency such that both parties need to understand the plan and the purpose. In some cultures, the grown children are extraordinarily involved in the business of the parents. Having spent almost twenty years practicing medicine in New York City, I have considerable experience with the most culturally and ethnically diverse population in the country, and perhaps the world. Add to that all of the multiple dialects from many of these countries and you begin to understand the linguistic and cultural complexity of dialogue that can exist between physician and patient, as well as the possible difficulties encountered during a prolonged treatment.

The need to tailor communicative techniques doesn't only apply to the different ethnic and cultural groups. How to explain a complex problem and outline an extensive cancer strategy varies even with different subsets of American society. A technique that I routinely employ is to use commonsense comparisons. For example, in the case of a patient who is an artisan—a person of technical skill such as an electrician or mechanic—there are various opportunities to explain disease and treatment strategies by using something borrowed from their daily life and, in doing so, to use common terminology. For instance, in the treatment of certain head and neck cancers, the surgeon might talk about an air bypass rather than a tracheostomy, a feeding tube bypass, rather than a gastrostomy, the windpipe rather than the trachea. The list goes on and on. By explaining in this manner, things become demystified and less frightening. I encourage doctors to continue to also use the medical words, but to offer the translation for their patients. Another effective technique is to refer to such procedures as a tracheostomy and a gastrostomy as "friends, not enemies, which allow us to work on your throat." In the management of the many cancers, there are hundreds of analogous examples. Getting these messages to the point of patient comfort is time consuming, and unfortunately, most busy doctors are short of this precious commodity.

If presented tactfully, such approaches enhance comprehension while showing respect for the patient's own expertise. There is, however, a fine line between making things understandable and condescension. Patients who are extraordinarily respectful and appreciative of a physician's education and dedication will also suffer slights and arrogance poorly. A person's dignity and pride must be respected. Importantly, a physician must avoid talking in florid proprietary lingo. The goal is not to impress, but rather to educate.

The legal profession is another segment of the population that benefits from extraordinary efforts at communication. I can speak with confidence on this subject because during the ten years in which I practiced at Georgetown University Medical Center in Washington, D.C., a substantial percentage of patients under my care were lawyers, many attached to the federal government. Some doctors shudder at the thought of caring for this population. Because of the issues pertaining to medical malpractice, a perceived antipathy has developed between these two important professions. Many physicians are defensive during their interactions with lawyers, worrying that the sword of litigation is automatically poised for the slightest variation from the standard. Conversely, many attorneys think that doctors despise them, and as a result, worry that they will not be cared for in the standard fashion. Neither of these suspicions is actually correct. On many occasions, I have had lawyers go to great lengths to reassure me by disavowing any connection with the litigation side of the profession. In point of fact, I have always felt that lawyers—even trial lawyers—are generally good patients, provided the physician is willing to devote the significant amount of time they require. Their meticulous analysis of explanations and facts, their need to do their own research, their need for multiple opinions, their need for the repetition of recommendations, and the general intensity with which they come to the physician's office, all reflect their training. From the very beginning of law school, lawyers are taught to think critically, to read and study all of the fine print, and to be cautious and generally skeptical. They have a hard time trusting people they don't know, including physicians. At a minimum, they may trust, but they usually want to verify, to paraphrase President Ronald Reagan. The search for multiple opinions often reflects this attitude. In dealing with lawyers, physicians must not be offended with this most fundamental of quirks. I am so reliant on trust in my dealings with patients that there is always an initial annoyance at what I sense as a failure on the part of a lawyer to trust what I am saying. My mature response, on the other hand, is to wait for the relationship to develop, and along with it the trust, just as with any other patient.

Lawyers are incessant note takers, and some doctors are unnerved by this as well as by their frequent request to record conversations. I have never felt this was inappropriate and have always encouraged patients to do whatever makes them comfortable in that regard. If going over our conversation by listening to a recording helps to achieve that, I'm for it. Otherwise, the chances are good that I would get a phone call in which the patient seeks to clarify what eluded them at the time of the office visit. In fact, being a big believer in eye contact between physician and patient, I would prefer that they record and pay attention, rather than spend time taking and organizing notes while I am explaining something to them. As has been said time and again in this book, to an experienced communicator, the countenance of a patient is usually revealing, and the eyes reveal so much of what is felt.

It is very common for a lawyer patient referred for management of a cancer to have done considerable research on their problem prior to the first office visit, and in the course of doing that, many that I have seen over the years have studied papers and other publications of mine on the particular topic of interest. I remember one humorous incident in which a young lawyer I was seeing for a benign tumor tactfully asked me why I had recommended to her what I did when in a paper that I had written fifteen years before I recommended a different approach. I was stunned at her level of knowledge, and after regrouping and realizing that it was a good question, I explained how during that time, the standard of care had changed. What I had recommended during both time frames—then and now—was consistent with the standards of the times. She was reassured, and the conversation went from there, but she did have some misgivings over the change—thinking, logically, that if the current method was correct, then the old method must have been wrong, and patients must have been the worse for it. I explained that "different" is not always better or worse, and that given the technologic development over the intervening years, the current standard was more practical in this particular situation. This very logical young woman accepted the explanation, and the treatment plan moved forward, during which I successfully removed the tumor. Once fully informed, she was a nervous, but a reasonable and very responsible patient.

The reason for telling this story is to point out that it is important that a physician not be threatened by such a challenge. Whether based on informational difference, or on what simply seems illogical, the question(s) are best dealt with in a nondefensive way. Modern information technology has created a world in which there is little proprietary information, and the computer savvy public of today is taking advantage of this fact more and more. The cancer doctor should be pleased, not threatened, by the informed patient. Admittedly, while patient research can be overdone, I believe it to be beneficial overall. I frequently have given patients a list of reading material when I thought they would be able to place what they would learn into proper context. I would much prefer that they read source material that I know to be authoritative, even if it is not exactly in agreement with my approach.

Admittedly, there is some downside to having a layperson reading the medical literature, especially that dealing with cancer. Within the medical community, and in that literature, opinions on diagnosis and treatment sometimes vary considerably. In fact, the differences do not reflect a right way or a wrong way but instead represent legitimate variances on how to do things, often with no difference in outcome. Cancer patients are discussed at tumor conferences, for instance, and disagreements among equally qualified physicians can, and frequently do, lead to different recommendations. These are often argued intensely. There is back-and-forth dialogue; egos are occasionally bruised; but usually, although not always, a consensus approach is finalized. This variability, whether in a conference or in the literature, can be disturbing to patients and can produce profound insecurity. While it is accurate to say that cancer treatment is and should be data based, and while there appropriately are standardized approaches to most cancers, the final decisions on what to do and when to it are based on a combination of judgment; timing; circumstances; the patient's state of health; and, finally, what is available and practical.

The availability of advanced technology is a common problem faced by those who practice outside of a medical center environment. Treatment strategy is thus tailored for the individual patient and illness, and also various geographic circumstances. I do not mean to contradict my earlier advocacy of patient education, but it must be understood that, in these circumstances, the time-honored cliché, "A little knowledge can be a dangerous thing," certainly applies. When decisions are made on the practical basis of what's available, rather than what's best, a patient's superficial probe into the literature can spark an understandable anxiety about the care he or she is receiving.

The antithesis of the behavior of lawyers is that of patients who are totally trusting, or who are so frightened that they do not want to be burdened with details and explanations. Overwhelmed patients will sometimes seek to place themselves totally in the hands of the doctors. For a patient to totally relinquish autonomy to a physician—without questions or doubts—might appeal to the doctor's vanity, but it is not a good way to start what is often a long and difficult journey. In order to make sense out of such blind trust of one's physician, one must understand the psychodynamics at work in the mind of a typical cancer patient.

Patients with substantial cancers are consistently terrified. Some handle and suppress their emotions more effectively than others, but with rare exceptions, fear stalks them. As a means of combating this relentless enemy, they often idealize their physician as a savior—and by doing so, they subconsciously are reassuring themselves. Vanity can be a seductive demon, and physicians possess the same personality flaws that make most people susceptible to it. Unquestioning faith is flattering but somewhat unrealistic. Since this book is partially designed to influence young doctors, this concept should be expanded a bit.

While we live in a social atmosphere in which the patient-doctor relationship is probably more egalitarian than in previous generations, and while it is safe to say that the medical professional has lost some of its glitter and perceived invincibility, much of the American public retains a fundamental belief that physicians are special. As with professional athletes, their star power as the academic elite is recognized early, and the deferential treatment starts then. By the time of medical school, the categorization happens in day-to-day life in which laypeople defer to the white coat; police, nurses, bill collectors, older people, and many others treat aspiring physicians differently; essentially they are enablers. Typical of that deference, I remember fondly the summer prior to starting medical school, I worked in an oil field as a "roust about" on an oil field crew. Initially treated in a guarded fashion, when my educational destination became known, I was called Doc, and was treated with great kindness and respect by a group of men with virtually no formal education. They were particularly worried about injury to my hands, and often my assignments reflected that fact. Like athletes, physicians grow up in a protected environment, such as I experienced in my oil field job, and that fact allows them to devote enormous energy and attention to their academic and clinical missions.

This protection is two-edged, however, and physicians tend to be emotionally and socially behind the curve as a result of it. Additionally, they evolve through a hierarchical system of residency training in which the higher the rank, the more numerous the minions, and of course the more the deference occurs. From there, the young physician is automatically welcomed into society, and in the office they are catered to. If they join a group as a junior member, they have to pay dues, of course, but in a solo practice, they reign supreme. At some point, most doctors mature enough to realize that this is not the real world, and that the rest of the workforce is not so privileged. Fortunately, most manage to keep their feet on the ground—expectedly, however, others don't. Vanity often accompanies deferential treatment, and that brings us back to the reason for going through this scenario—frightened patients can and often do appeal to that vanity in order to feel better about their own plight. This patient behavior is not always intentional; in fact, I am convinced that it is often primal and instinctive.

It should be noted that physician immaturity is not restricted to youth, and its perpetuation fosters egotism in some people as they age. This is especially true in the academic medical world, in which professorial status increases vulnerability to this most human of weaknesses. George Santayana wrote wisely in *Reason in Society*[1] when he stated "the highest form of vanity is love of fame." So when a patient or a family comes for consultation and says something like, "Doctor, we just want you to do whatever you think best, because we've heard you are the best there is," no matter how tempting it is to savor that "balm of adulation,"[2] a serious course correction is necessary.

While righting the situation, however, the physician should respond carefully, because overreaction in humility will often embarrass the person, or may even serve to undermine confidence in someone who so readily disavows excellence. I have usually handled this problem by resorting to humor: "You must have been talking to my mother—she always sings my praises," is my favorite comeback. Long after my dear mother had passed away, I continued to use her for this technique of neutralization; since her son the doctor could almost do no wrong, she certainly would approve being a party to this well intended deception. After this attempt at humor with the patient, I go on to explain that while I appreciate the compliment, its hard for anyone to claim title to "the best," since some surgeons are better at certain things than others, while not as good as some surgeons in other areas. In this way, one has not surrendered any claim to excellence or even denied being the best, but the patient has been led into a more realistic zone.

Patient care is obviously not always problem free. It is often said in the surgical world that a surgeon who denies having any surgical complications is guilty of one of two things: either not doing much surgery or lying. I cannot make the point strongly enough that the patient or family that has been allowed to remain in an unrealistic frame of mind can become bitter and angry when things don't go as planned. I have always taught residents to avoid what Merwin called the "collars and leashes of vanity,"[3] and never to allow such flattery to go unchallenged, lest they set themselves up for trouble.

I'm not immune to vanity, but in the academic world in which I have functioned throughout my professional life, the adulation of minions has been mitigated by smart, competitive people, all of whom have been encouraged and most of whom were willing to "challenge the professor"—sometimes less than subtly. Under such scrutiny, a wise person is disinclined to take himself too seriously. When such academic freedom does not exist, however, vanity goes unchecked, and the entire system suffers.

I have also been taught humility outside of the medical center environment, and I will leave this subject by telling a short tale of humor at my expense. A number of years ago, my wife and I were sitting at the Sunday dinner table with our young children and I told a silly, daddy-type joke—it might have been about why the rabbit crossed the road, or something equally ridiculous. I was taken aback when no one laughed. When I asked why no one had laughed at my joke, my then eight-year-old daughter—always the spokesperson for the children—responded with the straight faced and brutal honesty that only a child is capable of, "But daddy, we don't work for you, so we don't have to laugh . . . do we?"

· 19 ·

More on Physician Leadership: Being in Charge

$\mathcal{S}$ome of what is written in this book is based on interactions with patients and other health care professionals, and much is derived from my observations, successes and failures, and wisdom or lack of it. To a large extent what I have included amounts to a somewhat dogmatic method of managing cancer patients. So much of what I believe in this area involves character and interpersonal relationships. It's understandable that people use different barometers for judging character issues, but in my case, I have become more and more convinced that cancer patients who do not trust their physician's integrity ought to find a new physician. This is a theme repeatedly alluded to in this book.

In truth, it's important for the trust to be mutual, but the minimum ought to be the patient trusting the physician. I have always been sensitive to this issue, and when I even suspect that trust is marginal or absent, I'm troubled. If I detect this early and if it seems substantial, then I will try to find a graceful way of steering the patient in another direction, making certain that they are directed to a competent individual. If I believe the situation is repairable, on the other hand, then I usually confront the patient and the family, and while looking at them, say something like, "I want to make sure you understand and believe the things that I've told you. Even though I am not always right, I am always honest. I never lie to a patient. So if I seem encouraging, it's sincere." Often, I will go even farther by saying something in follow-up like, "You know, it's really important that you trust me, because when you think about it, can you imagine anything more dangerous than a dishonest surgeon? If you have the total trust that I'm talking about, and I don't mean sort of, but total, then you'll feel a lot more comfortable as we go along." Going even more into this blunt and simplistic monologue, I explain that things don't always go exactly as planned, and while what we do is usually problem free, certain complications can and do happen, despite our best efforts and most meticulous care.

A patient who has not received or who does not believe a realistic and thoughtful pretreatment explanation of the possibilities, bad as well as good, feels betrayed when things do go wrong. Patients have consistently amazed me with their willingness to accept complications and difficulties without anger or rancor when they believe in the forthrightness and integrity of their physician. When events do go wrong, the single most important response is for the physician to accept responsibility and to "play it straight" with people. Patients and families appreciate it when a physician expresses regret under these circumstances; however, first and foremost is the acceptance of responsibility.

Obviously, the time for talking about all of "the possibilities" with an operation or a treatment is not just before the actual treatment. Rather, such revelations and discussion in the early stage of the relationship give the patient and family time to absorb, reflect, and come back with questions. Not surprisingly, most people assume these things won't happen to them—that's okay—and because of this, once decisions are made, few seek to revisit the discussion about possible complications.

When talking to the cancer physician, especially a cancer surgeon, the patient's comfort level is influenced by a number of factors that evolve from the unspoken perception that the surgeon is in charge: the hospital chosen, the quality of the nursing, the operating room staff, and especially the anesthesia team, to point out but a few things on his/her radar screen. Most importantly, patients respond to a surgeon who is perceived to grasp and, in a sense, oversee the whole process, especially that pertaining to the actual operating room.

It's difficult for any anesthesiologist to deal with the fact that even though everyone shares in the responsibility for the patient's well-being in the operating theatre, the competence of the anesthesiologist—just as important as that of the surgeons—is essentially taken for granted. The patient usually does not have a relationship with the anesthesiologists or the nurses, and therefore, looks to their trusted surgeon (here's the trust word once again) to make sure everything will be OK. As the patient perceives it, in this setting the surgeon is the protector, or if you will, the patient's main advocate; and fundamental to what a patient seeks in a surgeon is strength without insolence, and calm without casualness. I have always told my residents in surgical training to take this issue seriously—develop peripheral vision, in which you notice everything that's going on in all activities of the operating room, from the time the patient is rolled in until entry into the recovery room. Whether justified on not, the surgeon will always be viewed as having some or all of the responsibility for most of what happens in this arena, bad as well as good. This somewhat sensitive subject involves the professional relationship between surgeon and anesthesiologist, and in order to explain it to nonsurgical people, I must review some of the relevant history of this part of the profession.

For many years, the general surgeon was a dominant figure in the profession. In medical centers, he (and in those days it was almost always a "he") controlled the surgical subspecialties, and not surprisingly, the management of the operating room, including anesthesiology. Anything that pertained to the operating room was within the dominion of the department of surgery, which was invariably chaired by a general surgeon. Essentially, general surgery reigned supreme! As medical specialization evolved, however, the chicks sought to leave the nest, and independent departments of anesthesia, urology, obstetrics-gynecology, orthopedics, otolaryngology, and others began to spring up. This revised pecking order should not reflect badly on general surgery because it was a reflection of decentralization and maturation of the profession—essentially no more than an organizational transition that most people feel is for the betterment of everyone, especially the patients. Each specialty sought autonomy, with control over their respective quality standards and training programs. Such was the case with anesthesiology, a fact that led to its independence from surgeons. So, as things have evolved, the "control" of the operating room and the standards within it have come to be regulated by anesthesiologists and surgeons of all subspecialties. What has evolved is a shared responsibility in which the patient's well-being, rather than the territoriality of the doctors, is paramount. It should come as no surprise to anyone, that there were some tensions between strong personalities along the way. As a result, it is no simple matter to discuss who is in control.

In the contemporary modus operandi, it is important for each of the operating room specialties to be in touch with what the others are doing, but that none exercise control over the others. Instead, shared influence is the path to environmental harmony in the workplace. Hence my contention that a surgeon must be engaged in all that happens in the operating room. It is the mark of an efficient team, rather than a lack of confidence, when the surgeon knows and understands what the anesthesiologist is doing, and vice versa. I am certainly no expert on what my anesthesia colleagues are doing, but I have always made it my business to try to respect what they do—to understand, ask questions, and most of all to be sensitive to the problems facing their team. The reader might ask how this relates to the patient's confidence in their surgeon's leadership. I refer you back to what I said earlier—that the patient looks to the surgeon for advocacy and protection, and if they are satisfied in that regard, overall confidence is enhanced.

The lack of a relationship between anesthesiologist and patient is not ideal and, in fact, works to the disadvantage of the former. This state of affairs should not reflect badly on anesthesia personnel, however, because it relates only to the logistics of operating room efficiency. In practical fact, a patient usually meets the anesthesia team immediately before the operation. This fact in itself serves to underscore the need for the surgeon to have engaged in a thorough preoperative discussion regarding the whole process, rather than only those issues that pertain to the actual operation.

With all of this in mind, it becomes obvious that a patient should be leery of a surgeon who shrugs his shoulders when asked about the expected involvement of the anesthesia team. Patients are greatly reassured by a forthright statement by the surgeon, such as "Rest easy Mr. Jones, I've worked with this anesthesia team before, and they're as committed to details and excellence as I am. 'We're' [the operative word] going to take really good care of you." Saying this may seem unnecessary, but hearing the words in the early stages of preparation for surgery and again just before the operation add up to major reassurance, no matter how brave the patient.

The interaction between surgeon and patient just before the operation should reassure and calm, not bring up scary facts. The surgeon should visit the bed-holding area where patients wait to go into the operating room. After a calm greeting with a positive expression to both patient and family, the surgeon should ask if there are any questions—if the proper groundwork has been laid in the office, the questions usually concern process, for example, "How long will the surgery take" or "Where should we meet you afterward?" Once this is concluded, I always make it a point to be in the operating room as the anesthesia team is preparing the patient. The role of the surgeon as the protector and advocate having been accepted, the last face that the patient should see before sleep should be that of their surgeon standing at their shoulder—hand on the patient's shoulder or arm, or even holding a hand, and importantly, making direct eye contact. A statement of reassurance at this time is good—"We're going to take good care of you, and I'll be sure to talk to your family right after the operation"—and the surgeon making eye contact is a peaceful additive to drifting off. With the modern drugs, all of these "little things" are barely remembered, but at a minimum, they seem valuable to me.

· 20 ·

Influences on Cancer Patients'
Attitudes and Receptiveness

$\mathcal{T}$here are many patient-related influences that affect the physician's effectiveness in dealing with a cancer patient—age, personalities, social circumstances, cultural factors, preconceived ideas, factual ignorance, superstitions, and an emotionally charged family atmosphere. Also, patients' imagination can lead them into an unpleasant zone—thoughts of illness, suffering, and death bring about erratic behavior. The very word *cancer* is terrifying, and no matter how illogical, for many people it is still thought of as a death sentence. In some such situations, once the word is uttered, mental blockage starts. The wise physician must anticipate and factor in all of these variables in dealing with patients.

THE ERA AND THE PATIENT AGE

I remember the secrecy that surrounded my grandfather's illness and death that resulted from lung cancer. He died at home in 1944 after a prolonged and painful decline. During those World War II years my mother, sister, and I lived with my grandparents, a common social situation in that time when many men were overseas. I witnessed my grandfather's decline on a daily basis, and the recollection of events is still clear. The instructions I had been given were carefully laid out. I was not to discuss his illness with anyone outside of the family, and the word *cancer* was never used, even within the household. In those days, cancer was viewed as repulsive and shameful, often not to be discussed—almost as if there was some form of guilt associated with it. Malignancies represented "rot and decay," the outward signs of which were humiliating. This was especially true of "female cancers," as they were referred to. Uterine, vaginal, and especially breast cancers led to an atmosphere of secrecy in which patients were shielded and hidden from public view and even sometimes from family. I have talked to many people who relate similar stories about the older members of their family. My wife's grandmother, for instance, died of breast cancer that she had discovered two years before actually seeking help. A combination of fear and shame had prevented her from doing so, and not until odor and bleeding made her secret untenable did she break her silence.

In today's world of openness and full disclosure, it's difficult to imagine such behavior in any segment of society; however, it was the norm rather than the exception as recently as the 1950s. The younger reader should not be quick to judge this as absurd, however, because until the 1960s the diagnosis was perceived to be a virtual death sentence. Even today, among the elderly of certain ethnic groups that are tied to older cultural ways, the mentality of secrecy and shame lingers regarding certain cancers. In the American mainstream culture fear of social stigma gradually loosened in the second half of the twentieth century, but even as late as the 1970s, these and many other personal matters were not openly discussed. The iconic figures of the times guarded such information intensely. This remained the status quo until First Lady Betty Ford and Ambassador Shirley Temple Black—two very public women—bravely used their breast cancers to introduce a whole new concept of public awareness and forthrightness with regard to this bane of women's existence. Since then, the publicity and public education regarding all cancers has become part of daily knowledge, and without doubt the modern attitude has saved countless lives. The present era and those to follow will be characterized by the growing knowledge of cancer's genetic mutations and familial propensities, and as a result, a whole new wave of enlightenment is before us. However, in underdeveloped countries, lack of public awareness, illiteracy, and superstitions are still enormous impediments to the achievement of modern health standards generally, and cancer standards, in particular.

As population turnover occurs, age as a generational encumbrance to patient self-advocacy is becoming less of a problem. Even though isolated pockets of superstition and myths from the past still exist in our society, the modernization of public thinking continues to grow. Another age-related matter, however, is of equal importance. A commonly held societal stigma associated with advanced age can cripple the self-esteem and resultant behavior of an elderly patient. The perception of older people is often based on esthetic and visual markers. Frailty, digital and vocal tremors, poor eyesight and hearing acuity, lumbering gait, and other products of age often belie an intuitive and keen intellect. The misinterpretation of these characteristics can lead an insensitive or thoughtless physician into a situation that is degrading and embarrassing for both patient and doctor alike. When such a misjudgment occurs, the doctor frequently remains uncorrected for a variety of reasons, such as the patient and family's desire to be polite or a sense of intimidation imposed by various artifices—hurried office personnel, white coats, the diplomas on the walls, for example. Unfortunately, patients and family usually do not complain about the offensive approach that assumes the elderly to possess marginal or no competence.

Often, the adult children bring their elderly parents to the doctor's office, and, given the acquiescence of the patient, it is entirely proper for the doctor to share everything with them. It is a fact, however, that doctors often talk around or partially exclude elderly patients in discussing their case with the son or daughter. Many older individuals welcome their children taking charge by making arrangements, transporting them, and being intimately involved in the conversation with the physician. However, such is not the case with others, who prefer autonomy and self-reliance. How to read and handle this situation varies, and the doctor's "people skills" and common sense need to be in play.

First and foremost, an initial appraisal of the environment prevailing in the examination room should judge the competence of the patient, no matter what their age. Many elderly patients have all of their mental faculties, and are proud to be their own advocate. I always start by focusing on and seeking the history from the patient, and as the response unfolds, I can judge whether or not to incorporate the children. It is far better to start with the patient and shift to the children than to do the opposite. On a number of occasions, I have walked into a room to see an elderly patient who is keenly aware and intensely independent of accompanying children, even resisting attempts by others to talk on his or her behalf. On the other hand, other elderly patients have greeted me with the admonition to talk mostly to the son or daughter that accompanies them. Basically, the patient should be the one who decides who takes the lead.

Most of us can recall stinging lessons learned in our youth. One such experience that is vivid in my memory was a turning point in my life regarding the topic of dealing with older patients. Having been out of surgical training a year or so—looking very young and probably acting a little cocky—I walked into an exam room in which two late-middle-aged women sat with their mother (I'll call her Ms. G.), who was the patient. She was almost 100 years old—ninety pounds and five feet tall at most—dark eyes and perfect teeth set in a cragged and wrinkled face that reflected not only advanced years but a lifetime of sun exposure, and a quiet demeanor that camouflaged a stormy self-reliance that I unknowingly was about to encounter. After introducing myself, I started out the questioning by addressing the daughters. I was about ten seconds into this when Ms. G. said, "Young man, I'm old, but I'm not stupid, and I certainly can handle this conversation at least as well as my daughters." In my embarrassment, I looked to the daughters, and one of them smiled and said, "We could have warned you, but you seemed to be in a hurry to get down to business." With that, I looked back at the patient's stern expression and she consummated her dominance by saying, "I'm still here, can we begin?" Lost for words, I meekly said, "Yes ma'am." Subsequently, I learned that Ms. G. had been a college professor; a successful author; by her choosing the sole occupant of her home; and, finally, entirely self-supportive. Her two daughters had been visiting, and Ms. G. had agreed to let them come along. I had simply not taken the time to analyze the situation, and had relied on those very flawed visual markers to which I referred earlier.

Later in my relationship with this patient—after several office visits and an operation that went very well—I returned to that embarrassing initial encounter and tried to make light of it, although I did offer an apology. She cut me no slack: "I accept your apology, but let that be a lesson to you." I often think fondly of this proud woman, and even though it is a humorous tale at my expense, I remain indebted to Ms. G. for "on the job training" and a valuable lesson. She has long ago passed on, but wherever she is, I wouldn't be surprised if she was still shaking her index finger at me.

THE SEARCH FOR ALTERNATIVE METHODS

Alternative methods of treating cancer are relevant to this overall discussion because on many occasions, patients or their families will ask about unconventional options, dietary supplements, or herbal remedies that they have heard about. The temptation to avoid harsh conventional methods can be strong. In this age of information technology, it's understandable that an intelligent person who possesses even modest computer skills would do homework on their problem, and in that capacity, they come into contact with the "alternative medicine" network that can open vistas of thinking dedicated to different methods of combating a variety of diseases, including cancer. In my opinion, it's important not to dismiss these possibilities out of hand, even though the physician has no real interest in incorporating them. Instead, we in the world of conventional cancer medicine should invite the patient's questions regarding the treatment plan to be used, and, while doing this, be willing to listen and explain the rationale for sticking with conventional methods. Often patients seek to feel involved in the battle. At a minimum, this can be psychologically therapeutic. It's time consuming to listen to and even sometimes read about what the patient is presenting as alternatives, and impatience can often lead to a dismissive attitude. Within reason, we should not allow such tedium to overcome our threshold of patience. I should confess, however, that as a surgeon, I usually deflect many of the alternative treatment questions to the medical oncologist on the cancer team because, as an internist, he or she is generally more knowledgable and more fluent with this dialogue.

Regardless of who is "answering the questions," and despite the need to always stay open to new ideas, it is important to keep in mind the fact that faddism and untested alternative methods not only can do direct harm but can also create delays in the employment of proven methods. In educating patients and to discourage them from chasing fantasies, the oncologist should make it clear that just because alternative or non-science-based methods work occasionally—or, conversely, just because standard, science-based methods can and do sometimes fail—this does not justify abandoning the discipline imposed by translational and clinical research methods.[1] Almost every aspect of cancer-related research and drug development is controlled by federal and state regulations that have been developed over the past few decades to protect the public from harm due to financial conflicts of interest in the research and pharmaceutical communities, inadequate patient protection in research studies, unsafe drugs and devices, and invasions of privacy. Even though founded on the best of intentions, many of the regulations have the unintended consequence of impeding the pace of new treatments; little wonder why frightened cancer patients who are aware of bureaucratic inertia and who are seeking to avoid the perceived misery of standard cancer care are vulnerable to the allure of alternative methods. Despite the shortcomings of the system, however, it is far better than the unregulated cancer care of many other countries.

To take one specific alternative methodology as an example, I point to traditional Chinese medicine. In urban areas with large Chinese populations, such as New York City, San Francisco, and others, this is much more than faddism, and the number of physicians practicing this ancient craft is significant. While this should not be dismissed, it should not replace data-based standard cancer care. Lest we be arrogant about this matter, however, we should keep in mind that the Chinese have relied on such herbal methods for thousands of years, and undoubtedly standard Western medicine can gain much useful information from this ancient culture. In the genre of cancer management, however, there is little room for variance, and we should adhere to data-driven standard methods.

Other alternatives that have sometimes been used in cancer management are strictly fads, totally lacking a scientific basis. During the course of my career, I have encountered cancer patients who, because of their rejection of standard methods, have sought a variety of advisors and helpers who employed holistic methods, macro-vitamin treatments, and many other unproven alternate treatments. I am reminded of the use of human interferon in cancer treatment. This was developed in Scandinavia in the 1970s by using pooled human blood. The development of recombinant technology in the 1980s as a source of interferon eliminated the dangers associated with viral contamination of human serum. However, until that breakthrough, one is left to speculate how often HIV and hepatitis viruses were spread by the administration of human interferon. Interferon was first directed to combat certain viruses, but within short order was randomly used in the United States on cancers that had proven resistance to conventional methods and even in some yet untreated malignancies. Another example of whimsical cancer therapy was seen in a number of patients who traveled to Mexico during the 1970s to receive drugs derived from cactus juice, despite a total lack of scientific evidence to support its use. The list goes on and on. Fortunately, the Federal Drug Administration has since followed a course designed to avoid the pharmacological frivolity that characterized those less-regulated times. More effective controls are now in place, and generally, there is a much more formalized approach to cancer management throughout the United States.

With all of this said, I believe that study and research into alternatives should be pursued. In fact, the medical profession has given credence to this area of investigation by creating an entire program of study of Alternative Medicine at the National Institutes of Health (NIH). I believe it to be a justified investment of taxpayer's money.

LANGUAGE AND CULTURAL ISSUES
AS THEY RELATE TO TRUST

There are overlapping themes between this section and the previous one, and I ask the indulgence of the reader for what I hope to be a minimum of redundancy. Depending on the geographic location, the issue of immigrant cancer patients who do not speak English is often no small challenge to the cancer team because of, among other factors, the unavailability of appropriate translators. In cities with large immigrant populations—New York, San Francisco, Chicago, Los Angeles, Miami, for example, different inner-city hospitals have substantial translation capabilities. For example, New York City's downtown hospitals (near Chinatown) have an abundance of Chinese translation capabilities, and in certain institutions even the signage and forms are available in both English and Chinese. In certain section of the borough of Brooklyn, Russian and Ukrainian translation services are available. When they are not, and when children or other relatives are utilized, inaccuracies in translation are often encountered. With the very serious cancer-related issues, this can be a huge problem. In diversified urban centers such as New York City, it is virtually impossible to provide translation services for all the languages. On several occasions over the years in which I practiced in New York, for instance, I operated on patients from Mongolia, and dealing with that dialect involved being totally dependent on the patient's children for translation.

Many years of practicing medicine in New York have introduced me to an amazing kaleidoscope of ethnicity. Although the scene is changing rapidly, the ethnic neighborhoods of this most international of cities are densely populated with Russians, Italians, Greeks, Poles, Asians, Latinos, Hassidic Jews, Africans, and many others, who retain their languages, religions, and culinary and other cultural traditions. Walking through such neighborhoods as Little Odessa or Chinatown—surrounded by music, smells, advertisements, dialects, and even dress of the mother country—gives one the feeling of being in the old world. This unchoreographed ballet of cultures known as the Big Apple is the quintessential reflection of the "nation of immigrants." On any given day, a rider on the subway might overhear five or six different languages. So when I hear people complaining about immigrants not speaking the "official language" of the country, I smile and am reminded that this has been a problem since colonial times. Until the unlikely discovery of a solution, physicians have to function, and in the world of cancer-related medicine, this is frequently problematic given the subtleties of certain important information.

In these ethnic communities the children, not surprisingly, are more Americanized, and they often accompany patients to translate, protect, and advocate for the parents. I generally have welcomed them into the exam room, at least while I take the history, and whether they stay for the physical examination depends on the patient's desire for privacy. When it is time to talk about the problem and the potential strategy to combat it, the children should be there, as long as the patient agrees. It is helpful if those present understand the doctor-patient discussion and also are supportive of the treatment strategy. This way, the disease and the plan of attack are discussed within the family after the visit, and patient understanding usually is enhanced.

It can be undermining, however, if the children are interested in a nonconventional approach. In such a circumstance, I always remind those seeking to advise that they assume an enormous responsibility by clouding the issues with nonconventional choices. I sometimes act as a parent to these children by saying that they should not assume the responsibility of advisor because with the likely failure of the alternative method, they will inherit an enormous sense of guilt. This is not an issue to be taken lightly. It's simplistic and naive for the doctor to take the approach that the family is "not the patient" and therefore, they don't warrant attention—often they are overly protective, involved, and profoundly influential in the family unit.

When family members, especially children, serve as translators for their parents, unless the physician understands the language being used, what the patient gets is often moderated into softer wording. In many cultures, the word *cancer* is anathematic and unmentionable. A humorous example of this is vivid in my memory. Once in the 1980s I was asked to see an elderly Italian man for what turned out to be a very curable head-and-neck cancer. In fact, the disease required only radiation therapy. Neither he nor his wife spoke English. Just as the translator and I were about to enter the examination room in which the man and his wife were waiting, two of their grown children cornered me in the hallway and respectfully begged me not to tell their father that he had cancer. Even though touched by this loving concern, I tried to explain the impossibility of hiding this from an adult. Not only was it unethical, but also impractical; how could I possibly talk about radiation therapy and other cancer treatments without revealing the real diagnosis? They gave me some wording that was well off the mark, and I told them that I'd see how things went, all the while knowing that what they asked was impossible. I politely sent them back to the waiting area and then entered the room. After a warm handshake, the first thing the man said in barely understandable English was "Doctor, please don't tell my children that I have cancer. I don't want them to worry." He had apparently learned how to form the words to make this crucial request, and that was the sum total of his knowledge of the language. I thought the mutual concern was all very sweet, even though dealing with all of the related intrigue caused me to fall far behind in my schedule that particular day.

While most of the younger generation of immigrants are Americanized as well as fluent in English, that is often not the case with their parents and grandparents. However, even in those who have achieved fluency in English, many of these older people come with preconceived superstitions and misinformation garnered in their country of origin. In many countries, medical standards are marginal and the esteem of the medical profession is low. It's almost axiomatic that an immigrant, whether fluent in English or not, will come under one of two headings: those that idealize, revere, and trust their doctor completely, and those that have virtually no trust and are inherently very suspicious. I mention this with specific regard to cancer patients because the various treatment strategies for this disease can be marathons of misery, both in body and in spirit, depending on what is used. Much is done that must be accepted on blind faith, and if a patient is dealing with a language barrier on top of fundamental skepticism, the misery index can be formidable. It has been my nonscientific observation that many of the immigrants from the countries of the former Soviet Union are untrusting of most authority figures, and have an especially hard time as this applies to medical issues. There are cultures in which all matters come down to how much money one can throw at a problem, and that broad stroke includes a lack of professionalism in the medical profession. For instance, on several occasions I have had families offer to pay me large advanced bonuses if I made a special effort to do a good job.

A unique culture, the Hassidic Jews in and around the New York City area, is socially and educationally insulated from the non-Hassidic world, and their primary language is Yiddish—a variant of medieval German. The combination of these factors creates a number of insecurity and trust issues for them. The key to the management of cancer patients from this subculture is the physician's communication with the rabbi of their particular synagogue. Usually schooled in many relevant issues and extremely influential in their community, the rabbi's concurrence does wonders in helping these very observant people accept and endure the treatment strategy.

Not infrequently, ethnically oriented families have large networks of relatives who are involved and filled with curiosity and concern. It can be extraordinarily time consuming for a busy cancer physician to deal with a crowd of ten or more people as if fielding questions in a press conference. I have known physicians who, in the interest of efficiency, have instructed such a group to confer among themselves and select a representative who is then given generous access to the doctor. The physician can then address the variety of questions in a fairly organized and often less emotional setting. If this method is introduced and handled tactfully and respectively, everyone benefits. Most often, a senior son or daughter is the designated person, but the doctor can give added respect to the parent with the specific question channeled through that spokesperson—"Does your mother (father) understand?" or "Does your mother (father) have any other questions?" This is usually done in front of the family, but even when such an inquiry is made in private, that deference to the parent becomes known throughout the family. Not only is it appropriate and respectful of seniority, it is effective in establishing a good working relationship with the family unit. Although this technique applies to other ethnic groups, it is especially effective in ethnic Chinese families, in which there is often retention of the ancient Confusion tradition of respect for one's elders.

As a result of having practiced medicine in New York City for years, I could fill many pages with tales related to this great American story of immigrants. As much as I would like to delve into that most enjoyable memory bank, I'll move on, and will conclude this section with a take home message: Even though culture diversity is very interesting and educational, dealing with it and its related issues in the practice of oncology can be time consuming and tedious. Therefore, this is not an arena for either a xenophobic or an impatient physician, and most of all, it is important to recognize and accept the fact that to a great extent we are the ones who must adapt. The cancer physician must never lose sight of the fact that these patients are almost always frightened, and such things as language differences heighten the fear factor. Imagine the totality of their situation—strange country, strange language, and a stranger for a doctor. Good communication is the oncologist's responsibility, not that of the patient. Even more important is the acceptance of the fact that real communication must include patient comprehension—and in the case of non-English-speaking patients, that means translation to their mother tongue. To paraphrase what I said earlier, if an aspiring oncologist is not willing to make these types of commitments, perhaps he or she should find another branch of medicine in which to practice.

IGNORANCE OF THE FACTS

Literally everyone, no matter how lacking in education, recognizes the word *cancer*. However, the general ignorance of and the lack of confidence in modern-day methods to treat it can sometimes be astonishing. I recall a situation—about eighteen years ago, if my memory serves me correctly—where I was a first-time guest on an all-male fishing trip with a group of very successful businessmen. We had had a wonderful day of trout fishing in an absolutely gorgeous Colorado stream—the food and drink made a perfect end to the day, and the men sitting around the table could not have been more interesting and enjoyable. One man, I'll call him Bill—a well-educated and very intelligent fellow, a combat veteran of World War II who was the quintessential example of the American success story—looked at me over his umpteenth glass of wine and said that he had been told that I was a cancer surgeon.

After I confirmed that, he stopped smiling and took on a challenging expression, whereupon I braced myself for an unfortunate story about a doctor's effort gone bad. "Now, doc," he said (up until then, I had been Roy), we've all had a nice evening, shared food and drink as a part of community and friendship, and since you now are certain that you are among discreet friends, you can tell us the real truth, can't you?"

"Absolutely," I responded, not knowing exactly what to expect.

"Isn't most of the data," he queried, "and most of the optimism about improvement in cancer treatment fabricated? Let's be real, a cure is the exception rather than the rule, right, and basically, you don't really expect to cure people?"

I was stunned, and started to respond as if to humor, when I realized that he was totally in earnest, albeit not quite sober. Looking around, I got no help from the group in dealing with this alpha male, so I tried only to rectify his state of knowledge. I got about thirty seconds into Cancer Treatment 101 when Bill politely interrupted to say that he had lung cancer, and his doctors had given him no hope. I tried my best to exit the conversation gracefully and without any more pontificating, but it was hopeless.

After a silent pause, Bill lit a cigar, and raised his glass to toast the excellent fishing of the day. He had not heard a word I said. End of attention span! End of subject! Period! Obviously, this is an extreme example used to make the point, but it is a true story, and if Bill even believed part of what he incorrectly thought, one can only imagine how many elderly people—less worldly—less intelligent, less educated, must be just as ill-informed. The fact that he had been diagnosed late in the disease may well have been related to inattention to his own health, and that may have resulted in his lack of faith in the medical profession in general, but he was beyond cure and in his mind that was the norm, rather than the exception.

Had I thought it would have served any useful purpose, and given the opportunity, I would have pointed out to Bill that most cancers, and especially lung cancer, are much more treatable than he described and, yes, curable when detected early in the course of the disease. Such is not always the situation, but in general, there is a linear relationship between time of diagnosis and survival. That is to say, the earlier, the better. Even more important, today we cure many cancers; of the almost 1.5 million new malignancies that are diagnosed in the United States each year, over 65 percent will be alive and well five years later. In fact, there are approximately ten million Americans living with a cancer history.[2]

Bill's story is not rare. I have talked to many elderly people about this issue, and am struck by how many are misinformed on cancer-related subjects. Admittedly, in this era of information technology, it has become less so, but ignorance and misinformation still are pervasive. As in Bill's case, there are complicating factors that help develop such a mind-set—his probable feeling of guilt for having smoked heavily for many years despite knowing better, and his lack of confidence in the medical profession, which probably partially resulted from the fact that, as I later learned, both of his parents and a sibling had died from cancer.

The experience with Bill was eye-opening for me, and I have since developed more tolerance and understanding not only for people's lack of knowledge but for the influences of life's experiences on their behavior and attitudes. Turning around that state of ignorance is a critical part of the job of the oncologist, and the money spent by the profession's leadership in its institutional outreach seems to be a wise and foresighted expenditure. Cancer prevention is obviously less expensive in the long run than is cancer care. Such sources as the National Cancer Institute database and various websites of organizations such as the American Cancer Society are more and more available to a public increasingly facile with computers.

Ignorance of the differences between chemotherapy and radiation therapy, as well as the preconceived notions and fears related to each, are common among the general public and especially in the elderly. It has been my observation that between the two, the image of chemotherapy suffers more. Historically, chemotherapeutic drugs were often viewed as agents of desperation invariably associated with hair loss, skin irritation, nausea, and vomiting; basically, with some exceptions, chemotherapy was thought to complicate rather than aid in the last part of life cut short by cancer. While there are still circumstances in which the administration of these agents is a challenge for the patient, the contemporary modus operandi of the sophisticated cancer team contains a medical oncologist (i.e., a chemotherapist) who accomplishes far more with less morbidity than ever before. Although a number of cancers are treated with plans that do not involve these agents, the cancer team discussions usually include the input of this important line of defense in the cancer war. It should be noted that a number of malignancies—certain sarcomas, lymphomas, leukemia, and others—are addressed medically, rather than with surgery or radiation, and chemotherapy or biologic therapy, the front line of treatment, cures many of these patients.

RELIGION AND LIFE AFTER DEATH

Sometime during the 1990s while I was practicing at Georgetown University Medical Center in Washington, D.C., I was asked to see a diplomat from one of the Middle Eastern countries. He was an educated and worldly man who had a head and neck cancer that required an extensive surgical operation to be followed by radiation therapy. The day of the surgery, I met with him and his wife in the holding area just prior to the scheduled operation. When I approached the bed, they were relaxed and had a pleasant greeting for me. No doubts, no hesitation, only a relaxed countenance in each. I remarked to him how calm he seemed, and he said to me, "I'm a devout Muslim, doctor, and I have put my life and your skills in the hands of God. Once that is done, I'll not worry because I know he will take care of me, and will guide you." I remember this vividly because it was so definite and sincere. He really was fine with the process, and really had turned himself over to Allah. At the time, I found myself envying that kind of intensity and faith about something so fundamental.

As I reflect on many years of caring for patients, I realize that such faith is not unique to Islam but can be found in all religions. It has been my experience that people with strong faith in the Deity and the associated afterlife generally are able to go through the cancer experience more easily than those who do not possess such beliefs. I say this as an observation, not a promotion, and undoubtedly one that will stimulate the disagreement of some; however, in my experience, this is unequivocally the case. Much like those patients who approach death comfortably because of a family support system, comforted by the immediate chemistry of love and friendship, the transition from life to death seems easier for spiritual individuals. Faith in a supreme being and an afterlife is the nuclear weapon of support for true believers. Many believe that they will be reunited with deceased members of their family, and in the mind of those with this belief, this reunion is actually what defines heaven. Others believe that to spend eternity with God is what defines that mystical place. Many devout people believe that life is merely a trial that must be endured in order to enter heaven, and therefore, in a sense, death is welcomed. In many, the only real negative aspect to dying is the separation from loved ones; otherwise, they are looking to something better than life on earth. If one studies history, people of medieval and other primitive times endured miserable lives, and looking forward to a better afterlife was completely understandable. Given the relative comfort of the developed contemporary world, however, it is a testimony of the power of spiritualism that so many continue to think of a better life after death.

Since it is my opinion that patients of intense faith handle the cancer experience better, I admit to having exploited this in my dealings with religious cancer patients. Without commenting on how deeply my own beliefs go, I will say that in those cancer patients and families that I thought to be religious, I have always encouraged them to look for spiritual help. Even though I never claimed to be such, I always let them think of me as religious if they chose to; and importantly, I never avoided the issue of spirituality. Many cancer patients will say "God bless you, Doctor." My response to this is "Thank you; God bless you too." Whether God hears such admonitions is somewhat uncertain in my mind, but what is certain is that such patients are comforted by it, and I have always felt that the use of these methods was well within my purview. I'm basically for that which helps!

According to a February 2009 feature article in *Time* magazine that was written by Jeffrey Kluger,[3] a growing body of scientific evidence suggests that faith may bring better health, and to quote one of the expert contributors to this article, Doctor Andrew Newberg, a professor at the University of Pennsylvania, "A large body of science shows a positive impact of religion on health." That the power of faith and prayer are applicable to the biology of cancer medicine seems to be somewhat of a stretch, and even more so to say miracles occur. That said, I should note that I have seen some amazing things in people who I thought had no chance to get well. Important to remember also is the rare but real occurrence of cancer's spontaneous remission. Not uncommonly, tumors cease growing and exist in a relative state of dormancy for years.

Whether the result of the body's immune system, an aberration of tumor biology, or the miracle that many religious people firmly believe in, the reader is urged not to automatically label these events as the quirky fantasies of religious fundamentalists. The following are just a few of the research institutes devoted to studying the association of religion and medicine as their main focus: Center for Spirituality and the Mind, University of Pennsylvania; Center for Spirituality and Healing, University of Minnesota; Center for Spirituality, Theology and Health, Duke University; and National Center for Complementary and Alternative Medicine, National Institutes of Health. There are a number of very intelligent scholars who are studying the body's physiologic link to spiritual forces, and as with all alternative approaches to human disease, we should offer support and sustenance to such investigations. While doing so, however, we should continue the implementation of standard, science-based cancer evaluation and treatment. Because knowledge begets more knowledge, molecular biology and genetics have fostered a scientific revolution that is probably only the beginning of a period of exponential intellectual growth. The knowledge of the neurochemistry that links the brain and disease is still in its infancy.

QUALITY OF LIFE CONCERNS AND THE SEARCH FOR AUTONOMY

To some patients, the loss of what they value in their everyday life in an effort to be cured of a malignancy is an unacceptable trade off. Even if a cure is highly likely, they opt for quality rather than quantity of life. This is not a modern concept; certain Roman philosophers believed that it was more important to have lived well than to have live a long time.[4] As a means of emphasizing this point, I have often related the story of a patient I will call Mr. C., whom I first saw in 1983, when I was a surgeon on the Head and Neck Service at Memorial Sloan-Kettering Cancer Center in New York City. He had a fairly advanced laryngeal cancer, which by the standard of care in 1983 required a total laryngectomy and postoperative radiation therapy. While that treatment package was curative in a high percentage of patients, it would have irreversibly altered his ability to talk, and would have required a permanent opening in his trachea. Mr. C. was the quintessential urbanite—a cultured and refined New Yorker. When I told him the "good news," the high probability of cure, he smiled and said, essentially, "thanks, but no thanks." He was willing to try radiation therapy alone, but nothing else.

This dignified older man proceeded to tell me that he and his wife were childless and that their very pleasant life consisted of his activities with the Metropolitan Opera, the theatre, his academic lecture schedule, and their very busy social life among the intelligentsia in the galleries and museums of New York City. All things considered, he and his wife had decided that the quality of life issue outweighed all else, and that if we couldn't find a more acceptable way, he didn't want to live, and in fact, would "take care of his own arrangements for the end." This suicide threat was not even subtle, and I thought that his courteous smile surely belied what underneath was a desperate and depressed man. Such was not the case, however, and the cool demeanor and steely resolve of this chilling statement unnerved me. When I turned to Mrs. C. for help, she stood up, walked over to her husband's side, rested her hand on his shoulder, smiled, and by her countenance confirmed that, indeed, she was on board with this plan. I then played my trump card by saying that if we used radiation alone, there was little chance of cure, and a few months down the road, we would be back to the same place, except that the chance for cure through salvage surgery would be much worse. He countered by saying that surgery at that point would be no more acceptable then it was presently. Therefore, my statement was moot. I did not make the point that a death from uncontrolled laryngeal cancer was a most unpleasant and prolonged way to die. He had already negated that argument with his plan for ending his own life, rather than face all of that.

"We understand all of this," said Mr. C., "and we would never hold you responsible for failure. This is what we've decided, and this is what we want. Will you arrange it and remain our doctor, after the treatment? We trust you completely, and by the way, there's no need for you to suggest a second opinion; you are the second opinion."

After my own adjustment to the patient's firm resolution in totally ignoring me, I went along with what they requested. The patient was treated with radiation, did continue on the board of the Metropolitan Opera, and did continue their lifestyle for some time to come. I received Christmas cards from the Mr. and Mrs. C. for over ten years, and on each card was the picture of a dapper couple, dressed to the nines, and a sweet note wishing my family and me a happy holiday. The "PS" that was always at the bottom noted the number of years since we had treated his cancer "his way." I never interpreted this as sarcasm, but instead chose to let it remind me that sometimes the patient knows best and that one should follow the age-old rule of thumb, "Doctor, listen to your patient—it's often good advice." It's worth noting that at the time of this writing—twenty-six years later—the standard of care for Mr. C.'s cancer is, in fact, not laryngectomy but radiation therapy. I have often wondered if Mr. C. had proprietary information in 1983.

There is a measure of maturation in a surgeon's willingness to deal with the situation that I have just cited with Mr. C., and I might add that my interaction with him was one of those significant educational situations in my own maturation. I was really frustrated by his quiet determination to ignore my advice, no matter how strongly I made the case. I couldn't believe that his final answer was "thanks, but no thanks"! My inclination was to let him find a radiation therapist, and take no responsibility for his care. Instead, I reluctantly yielded, referred him to the proper radiation oncologist, and arranged to stay involved and see him in follow-up along with the treating oncologist. The rest is history.

The message here for young oncologists is not so much the fact that the patient turned out to be right and I was wrong (by today's standards), nor is it not so much that he sought the correct treatment for the wrong reasons. What is important is that after considerable research and contemplation, he and his wife decided that the recommended treatment was worse than the alternative—which in his case was a planned suicide. This was clearly an educated and intelligent patient—levelheaded and not depressed—insisting on autonomy.

Other patients encountered in my own career—a diplomat, a network television newscaster, a noted Broadway star, a TV network president, an accomplished movie actor—also simply would not accept substantial surgical procedures that would cripple their speech and voice or disfigured them. Mr. C.'s reasons for saying "thanks, but no thanks" related to the potential inability to socialize within his cultured and sophisticated network. In the case of these other patients, it was all about refusing career-ending treatment. More often than not, their choice of treatment failed, but in these, there usually were no regrets.

No matter how strong the physician's competitive instincts to defeat the disease, in the final analysis the decision should be made based on what is best for both the patient's physical and psychic health. To put it another way, what we do should be about the patient, not about the physician. The patient's reasons for going in this direction are essentially irrelevant. If they still feel the same after the facts have been bluntly laid before them, so be it. I have had a long and busy clinical career, and reflecting back brings to mind a number of cases similar to those that I have cited in which the patient has said "thanks, but no thanks"; this is not a rare happening.

The whole patient autonomy concept has taken on a life of its own in the current era of widely distributed information, advocacy groups, and patients who do their homework. With today's patient population, the physician's proclamations are not necessarily accepted as gospel, and the youth of the profession must accept, and those of my generation must adapt to, this permanent alteration of behavior in the world of medical care. I can remember a number of very radical operations and treatment plans that I imposed on patients in the past, and as I think back, I confess that knowing then what I know now, in some of them, I would not have recommended what I did. Even more revealing with my self-appraisal, I would now not accept for myself what I did to them. I have discussed this matter with other senior surgeons who share my feelings that in the past we did not always pay enough attention to patient quality of life. In the contemporary cancer care world we should be committed to the goal of maximizing the chance for cure while maintaining a strong emphasis on the individual's quality of life. Curing the cancer at any cost—that is, returning the patient to society, cured but incapacitated—is no longer an automatically accepted strategy, and the approach should always be sternly challenged. Strategies of organ preservation and function are, therefore, constantly being developed and utilized in the oncology world of today.

During the twentieth century, surgeons appropriately pushed limits, all the while seeking to perfect bigger and bolder operations; what has been achieved is truly remarkable. Even though we have always sought enlightenment and knowledge, this emphasis on surgical elegance has dominated us largely for lack of scientifically based alternatives. That is, however, no longer the case. By and large, we are now appropriately focused on multiple methods of combating cancer. It should be noted that although the U.S. Food and Drug Administration has yet to approve a therapeutic cancer vaccine, a number of experimental vaccines are making their way through clinical testing. Vaccines for melanoma, non-small-cell lung cancer, non-Hodgkin's lymphoma, HER 2 positive breast cancer, renal cell carcinoma, glioma, prostate cancer, acute myeloid leukemia, head and neck cancers related to human papillomavirus (HPV), and others are currently in Phase I, II, or III trials. Where all of this will ultimately settle is uncertain, but my speculation would be that future cancer treatments will utilize combination methods—surgical, chemotherapeutic, biologic, and nuclear—on a routine basis, and as genomic research evolves, prevention and alteration will surpass much of what we do today.

SEXUALITY AND OTHER SOCIAL MATTERS

In some respects, my thoughts on how cancer influences patient sexuality could have been blended with those in the preceding section concerning general quality of life issues. In most, this pleasurable slice of life's experience can continue, despite having to share the stage with that villain called cancer. At a minimum, the exploration of sexuality by the cancer patient doesn't necessarily have to be abandoned. That is, of course, with the understanding that the gold standard of sexuality is the level that one has achieved prior to the introduction of the cancer distraction—no more!

The treatment of malignancies of the sex organs and adjacent areas, as well as certain endocrine glands—prostate, perineum, penis, testicles, vagina, ovaries—obviously have a direct impact on sexual performance, some to a greater degree than others. Treatments of other cancers, while not causing a direct compromise of sexual capability, can create embarrassment and self-consciousness that leads to a huge compromise of a person's self-esteem and sexual life. Such is seen with breast cancer treatment; colon cancers in which there is a need for a colostomy; various head and neck cancers that require disfiguring surgery (jaw and tongue removal, laryngectomy, gastrostomy, and tracheostomy tubes); limb sarcomas that require amputation; and many others.

These are identifiable physical problems that can alter a patient's sexuality. Beyond these factors, however, are the subtle and intangible matters that compromise a person's sex drive—such things as alteration of smell and taste; xerostomia (dry mouth); esthetic compromise related to loss of hair, breasts, and muscle mass; depression; fatigue; anxiety; and insomnia, to name a few. Erectile dysfunction, and in both sexes the general loss of sexual appetite, are not small concerns. In their popular source book for patients, *Choices*, Morra and Potts point out that since a substantial percentage of the general population has sexual problems caused by stress, it's certainly understandable why cancer and cancer treatments might change sexual relationships.[5]

The quintessential example of cancer's intangible impact on sexuality is seen in females with breast tumors. For better or for worse, in our culture, breasts epitomize femininity. Sexual allure, lovemaking, infant nursing—all of these are equated with womanliness, and the breasts are a focal point in each. The time in which radical mastectomy was casually employed is mercifully past, and the esthetic impact of breast operations has been substantially mitigated by the skills of reconstructive surgeons. Despite these advancements, the discovery of a breast mass is frightening, even though it is common knowledge that the majority turn out to be benign. Such a finding evokes multiple issues and emotions, many of which are unrelated to cure. This topic is the subject of much literature, and no more than a cursory mention seems indicated here, but these issues are relevant to the mission of many oncologists, and guidance into the right support system is a primary concern for the entire cancer team.

In doing research for the development of this book, I interviewed a number of women survivors of this disease, and I was struck with the difference of attitude relative to age. Not surprisingly, older women were less concerned about the implications for their sexuality and zeroed in more on the cure issue. What did surprise me was that several women confessed that following the treatment of their cancer, they had sensed in their partner a very subtle primordial change—not so much a lack of sexual attraction, but a concern or a feeling of avoidance of disease. They sensed in their partner a fear of contagion. One woman said she felt like "untouchable goods." It's interesting to speculate about whether this feeling that these women confessed to was only a product of their imaginations, but I must say that those that related this feeling were intelligent and perceptive, and not individuals prone to hyperbole.

When I first encountered this most private of thoughts, my first inclination was to dismiss it as an ill-perceived notion; surely no intelligent partner could be concerned with the contamination of their own body by cancer. However, I am reminded of a time in the not too distant past when people with oral cancer queried me about transmissibility to their partners, and I might add, on several occasions, their partners asked me privately about their own safety. My dogmatic response at the time was a resounding no—there's nothing to worry about. Since then, we have learned of the human papillomavirus and its carcinogenic capabilities—first in the uterine cervix, and more recently in the oral pharynx. As a result, the dogma of the past must be altered to consider the possibility of oral-genital and genital-oral transmission of this carcinogenic virus—sexual transmission. I say this so that the reader is not dismissive of the fact that some partners may have a sense of personal fear to which they would perhaps never admit but which is well within the perceptual capability of a woman keenly in tune with her mate, and additionally, who already has concerns about the impact of her breast cancer on her personal appeal. I make no attempt to guide the reader in understanding these complicated psychological issues. Instead, I seek only to alert them to their existence and to point out the consistent need for comprehensiveness in dealing with cancer patients, no matter what their sex, no matter what the type of cancer. This is not work for the shortsighted dilettante who may be technically elegant, but ignorant of the big picture.

On repeated occasions in this book I have mentioned the benefits of a doctor touching and making physical contact with a patient. So it is with cancer victim and partner. I am convinced that most humans gain solace from being touched, and being in a relationship should provide ample opportunity to indulge this most human of needs. It is my impression that much of the sexuality needs of the cancer victim and partner stop short of actual sexual intercourse. Instead, the comfort afforded by caresses and other expressions of affection are important for both partners, regardless of who is afflicted with the disease and undergoing treatment. In a sense, having cancer is a provocative experience—not only of anger, but also of sadness. The spiritual impact of love and concern is especially relevant to the one who has the cancer. Anger is more of an individual matter, and working that emotion out is accordingly more of a singular endeavor. On the other hand, sadness can and should be shared.

Doctors are often uncomfortable having this dialogue with cancer patients, and if such is the case, I suggest referring the patient and their partner to a sex therapist or a psychotherapist who works with couples. Those therapists who are well trained usually belong to one of the two following organizations: American Association of Sex Educators, Counselors and Therapists; and National Association of Oncology Social Workers. Additionally, the American Cancer Society is an organization replete with resources for advice and counsel.

• *21* •

Communication When There Is Still Optimism for Cure

$\mathcal{O}$ccasionally, a patient will question the physician about the process of death, even though the cancer is treatable or likely curable. This is a highly variable situation, with some patients being afraid to ask for fear of hearing what they fear most. Some will be satisfied with limited information, and to them delving into all of the negative possibilities is not useful. Obviously, with cancers in which the outlook is optimistic, the conversation is slanted differently—upbeat but realistic.

Even in this group of patients, however, there are requests to talk about death. Some thoughtful and compulsive patients want to plan their lives by knowing all the possibilities, bad as well as good. The honesty of this particular discussion is important, and the patient's confidence and trust in the forthrightness of their physician is enhanced by a realistic and serious response, rather than the patronizing banality of unfounded reassurance. In this situation, I rely heavily on probability and statistics to explain the potential for various outcomes. There are those of my colleagues who disagree with this approach. I know oncologists who never quote statistics, and instead talk in terms of a "good or low chance," or "a high likelihood." Peter Ubel, a professor of medicine and psychology at the University of Michigan, has recently been paraphrased in an article in the *Annals of Internal Medicine* as advocating clear and simple facts for patients to contemplate, but he discourages physicians from using percentages to describe treatment effects and survival.[1] He believes that many Americans do not comprehend information presented in this way. His research suggests to him that visual aids—bar graphs and pictographs—convey the information more effectively.

Earlier in this book I admitted that my advocacy of certain theories, concepts, and methods in dealing with cancer patients and their families were not sacrosanct but were merely what works best for me. In this regard, others should use what is most effective for them. I have great faith in the well-spoken word, and I feel more confident in my ability to communicate without reliance on graphic aids. I often use diagrams of anatomy and, on occasion, even bring out a human skeleton for educational purposes. However, when talking about cure, survival, and the probability of each, I would rather make eye contact and talk in an understandable manner not compromised by visual distractions.

When statistics are used, it is important to qualify them by not talking in bland quantitative jargon. In other words, it is possible to present the "fifty-fifty chance" as a glass that is half full, rather than half empty. The physician should lead the conversation to the positive, rather than the negative. Allow me to give a specific example: For certain vocal cord cancers, the likelihood for cure is about 90 percent after either radiation or a larynx-sparing surgical procedure. The way I would approach such a patient is with an added portion of optimism by pointing out that if we start with a nonsurgical approach, nine out of ten patients will be cured. Patients seem to be more reassured with this than referring to 90 percent. If they are the unlucky one in ten who fails the front line of treatment, then we can use the surgical procedure as a second line of defense. In this situation, there are still eight out of those ten patients that failed radiation in whom the voice-sparing operation will cure the cancer. If one does the math, this sequence of treatment options adds up to an almost certain cure. The patient would be told that while guarantees are never wise, the overall outlook with this approach is hugely optimistic. Some patients even go so far as asking, "OK, but what if the second line fails also?" I would then tell them that there is a third line of defense that is quite effective also, although the price involves a total laryngectomy, with the subsequent loss of normal voice. I strongly emphasize the extreme improbability of this full scenario occurring, and to further focus on the positive, I point out that in the unlikely event of losing the larynx, the natural voice is forfeited, but with a simple reconstructive procedure, communicative skills are restored, and life can go on.

In the case of a less favorable malignancy, while it is often possible to emphasize the positive, one cannot and never should hide from the truth. For example, with a cancer in which the overall prognosis is a 40 percent likelihood of survival, if the patient's particular tumor is of an earlier stage, or if the individual morphologic features of this particular tumor are more favorable, spending time educating them about stage and morphologic-related factors can often give the patient encouragement without deceptive or false hope. The simple fact is that different patients' immune systems handle tumors differently, and this particular patient might be more likely to be part of the 40 percent than the 60 percent. In effect, with this technique, we have de-emphasized the 40/60 data and if nothing else, given the patient the perception that he or she is probably on the left side of the ratio. With that perception automatically comes the implication that the outlook is actually better, at least in this particular case.

While seemingly simplistic, this "emphasis alteration" is factually honest and gives a patient something positive to hang on to. It is my contention that people relate better to the spoken word of explanation and encouragement than to the visual representation of probability. In all of this, there must be a core of honesty, however, and to return to a recurring theme in this book, deception by false encouragement has no place in any of these discussions. So when the prognosis is bad, one cannot hide from the truth, but unless it is hopeless, the doctor should always try to find some means of encouragement.

I keep coming back to the theme of physician honesty and patient trust, and in doing that, I ask the reader to indulge me, rather than yawn. My intention is to promote the realization that this human formula may be the common denominator for most of what we do in dealing with cancer patients. It's easier to convince someone to look at the bright side and to find hope if they believe their physician would never falsely encourage them. In conversations in which I am talking to patients about their prognosis I reinforce this atmosphere with added techniques. In the hypothetical tumor with the 40/60 percent issue, once the "emphasis alteration" is introduced to the patient, I often conclude with a straightforward statement while leaning in close and making direct eye contact: "It's important," I say, "that you realize that I haven't exaggerated in this discussion—you can believe what I've told you. I'm not always right, mind you, but I never give false encouragement to a patient. You believe this, don't you?" Depending on the patient's personality, I will frequently make physical contact while I am saying this. Resting a hand on a man's forearm, or with a female patient, actually holding her hand while making this direct statement can be a powerful combination that provide solace, trust, and hope to frightened cancer patients. I cannot emphasize enough the importance of three things—eye contact, directness of speech, and the laying on of the hands. Obviously, some people do not like to be touched and some feel as if "their space" is being invaded when a doctor gets physically close to them. One has to judge a patient's body language on an individual basis.

I want to pass on one more "personal technique" that I have used for years in an attempt to reassure. When the office consultation is done, if time permits, it is helpful for the doctor to accompany the patient out the exam room and into the hallway, all the while putting an arm around a shoulder or holding an arm. If the family is present, it's important to focus on the patient for this exit reassurance. While walking a few steps at the patient's side, the doctor is able to talk softly and intimately, "I know you're worried, but we'll be with you the whole way and keep you informed; and I promise, we'll take very good care of you. We pay a lot of attention to details." These last two points are especially reassuring to a patient who is facing surgery.

Finally, I want to make the case for "laying on of the hands." Most patients do like to be touched, and the physician who understands the subtle methodology of this very human need doesn't come off as paternalistic or too familiar, but instead exudes a welcomed warmth and confidence. When the chemistry is good with a particular patient, one can almost feel the flow of communication at the "touch point." Finally, some patients are often emotionally moved to the point of seeking to hug or even kiss the doctor. Some doctors are uncomfortable with such intimacy, but for most a warm and open receptiveness to a physical overture like this is entirely appropriate. Importantly, this demonstrativeness does wonders in establishing a deeply founded physician-patient relationship. Obviously, the initiation of such gestures must come from the patient. Later in an established and trusting relationship, a hug and/or a kiss are frequently exchanged with patients, and it is especially interpreted as sincere and well founded when it is done in front of family—spouse included. But the physician must be very sensitive to a patient's capability for such social intimacy and must always take care to avoid that which is repugnant or uncomfortable to the patient. Some people are raised in homes where physical demonstrativeness is nonexistent. I know physicians who would not think of engaging in such activities as I have described—they don't even do so in their own homes. On the other hand, some homes are full of constant physical contact. My maternal grandmother, for instance, hardly would allow her grandchildren to cross the room without giving her at least a peck on the cheek. The point is that, as in most new relationships, the physician should size up the personalities early on, and the approach should be tailored accordingly.

Another way of encouraging patients and helping them find hope is to point out the ever-changing and growing research efforts that might be going on with the particular cancer in question. While it is a bit of a stretch to encourage it, some patients like to hope that there may be something on the immediate horizon that will be useful for them. Encouragement can also be given, particularly for a patient in the posttreatment stage, by discussing the bell-shaped curve of disease recurrences, showing how they usually happen in the first one to two years after treatment. The farther that a patient progresses on the horizontal axis, the time line, the less likely is the chance for a recurrence of that particular cancer. In this way, a patient has reason to be increasingly encouraged as time passes. One tumor-free month follows another, and as the momentum of encouragement builds, so too does their emotional strength. This method should not be launched, however, until the down slope of the graph is reached. Whether this is psychotherapy or merely positive reinforcement is irrelevant. In my experience, it works!

Putting a patient in touch with support groups and health projects can also encourage and help to build hope. Even though activities such as exercise and dietary programs are probably not actually helpful from an oncology standpoint, they represent a combative participation in fighting the disease. Participants feel better for taking part in their welfare, so to speak. I have found this to be particularly helpful in patients who have been victimized by cancers that relate to lifestyle, such as aero-digestive cancers, in which smoking, drinking, and dietary factors play an important role.

It is essential that through all of this the physician not abdicate leadership as the alpha member of the support team. While support groups and other team members are immensely helpful in the ongoing encouragement of the patient on their way to cure, the cancer physician must remain sensitive to the emotional ties that a treated patient feels. Whether the treatment is successful or not, those ties remain strong and dependent. Once an oncologist has accepted this role, he or she owns it. This point is driven home by seeing the consistent distress of even cured patients upon the retirement of their cancer physician. I went to great lengths to counteract this when I retired from active practice, but many emotional patients—despite understanding the inevitably of the passage—made the separation difficult for them and for me.

· 22 ·

Communication Once
Treatment Failure Is Obvious

$\mathcal{N}$ot uncommonly, when it becomes obvious that the treatment has failed, the patient and family feel anger toward the medical team; however, with a mature response to this emotion, the doctor is usually able to make the point that the cancer, not the cancer team, is the enemy. The key to overcoming this initial response to failure is a trusting and affectionate relationship with the patient and family established well in advance of death—generally, starting at the time of the first office visit. The building blocks of enduring trust start early and are based on a number of factors: having correctly identified the enemy and having established a doctor-patient alliance in the fight against the enemy ("we are in this together"); the continued nourishment of the partnership by physician availability; consistent compassion and sincerity; and finally, the comfort of the patient and family in knowing that they will not be abandoned, no matter the outcome.

Lest the reader underestimate the importance of this last thought, I should say that when dealing with cancer, the most deeply felt component of the physician-patient relationship is trust—not just in the truthfulness of the physician but, just as important, in the confidence that he or she will be there until the end. It is an understatement to say that a pervasive fear—sometimes subliminal and sometimes overt—of most cancer patients is the fear of being abandoned. On many occasions, I have felt my own inadvertent emotional separation occurring when I realized that a patient's situation was hopeless. As I will illustrate, there are occasions when one begins to pull away without even realizing it. It is also common for the cancer team members to begin the process of emotional detachment as death approaches.

As a means of separating this from the theoretical, I interviewed a number of families of deceased cancer patients, and many—not a random few—remarked how they had felt the oncologist had emotionally withdrawn from their loved one as the end approached. I believe that these are usually unintentional slights and don't represent insensitivity. Instead, they are understandable human instincts spawned from self-protectiveness. No matter how understandable, however, all members of the team, especially the lead oncologist, must be vigilant not to let this happen; the dying and their families are keenly sensitive to this particular tendency.

Late in my career, a delightful nineteen-year-old woman (I'll call her Judith), was referred to me for treatment of a high-grade salivary gland malignancy. Despite the lack of evidence of metastasis, her prognosis was guarded because of the natural history of this particular type of tumor. Judith was frightened but optimistic and filled with idealism and hope, and the intimacy and love between her and her accompanying parents was something to envy. In fact, she reminded me of one of my own daughters—that alone led me to an almost instant bond with her. The cancer strategy was outlined in an upbeat conversation—surgery followed by postoperative radiation therapy. Everything went without a hitch, and even ten months later, there was no evidence of disease; all seemed well. In the meantime, I had come to a state of real mutual affection with the whole family. Their emotional Italian dealings with me were loving, demonstrative, and filled with heartwarming hugs, small presents such as food, and things for my wife—you get the picture. Judith had gone back to college and was moving on with the verve of youthful optimism.

The sudden thunder of realization came, however, at the one-year visit, when lung metastasis was detected. It would seem that we had won the head and neck battle, but the lung metastasis heralded almost certain overall defeat, given the fact that there was no effective drug for this particular type of tumor. Giving up was not on her agenda, and during the ensuing year in which chemotherapy was given, this young woman repeatedly demonstrated extraordinary courage. She comforted her parents, and even periodically gave her doctors a pat on the back for encouragement. When the relentlessness of the cancer became obvious, in an attempt to respect her adulthood, I sat with her and talked about death and dying. This young woman was intelligent and, as it turned out, had not been deceived by blind optimism. I proceeded to assure her that I would be with her until the end. Judith died some months later, surrounded by those she loved—cachectic and exhausted—but still of brave countenance.

The point of this story is to confess two things: First, the chemotherapy made her feel terrible, and the whole medical team knew it would be ineffective. Perhaps we should have let her get the most out of the last part of her life unencumbered by nausea, hair loss, and other unpleasantness. Second,

as I look back on that time subsequent to the discovery of disease recurrence—when the course was clear—I realize that despite my awareness of
the tendency to emotionally pull away, and despite my admonition in this
writing to guard against doing so, in this particular patient, that's exactly
what I did. I tried hard to compensate and cover up the inexorable force of
self-protectiveness that was having its way with me. This young woman had
easily found residence in my heart. When she died, my wife grieved with me,
since she knew the whole story. We attended the wake,[1] which was on Long
Island. The greetings were as one might expect—emotional and tearful. During an embrace, Judith's father told me how glad they were to see me, because
they had sensed that I had separated from them, and that, perhaps, I didn't
feel the same as before. My attendance, and especially the accompaniment of
my wife, had reaffirmed their daughter's importance to me.

Aside from the guilt associated with the accuracy of their instincts, I
was blown away by the realization that the family—and almost certainly the
patient—had sensed that which I did not even realize myself. I was reminded
of the importance of my original commitment to the patient and the family. They really had heard what I said many months before about my staying
power. More than any other of my experiences, this story verifies the fact that
the dying and their families are keenly sensitive to doctors' human instinct
to pull away out of self-protection. As I reflect on all of this, it is sobering
that after all of the years of caring for cancer patients and after so many death
experiences, I was once again forced to come to grips with the extraordinary
weightiness of my life's work.

The notion of the cancer team doctor remaining in attendance until
death is obviously an ideal, and when geography allows it, there does exists a
solemn responsibility for that doctor to remain in attendance if in the hospital, or in touch if at home or in a hospice, until death. The practical implementation of this is not always possible, however, because cancer patients are
often referred from their hometown setting into an urban medical center for
treatment. When this is the circumstance, the local physicians have to do the
best they can with the resources available.

As our sophistication in cancer management has matured, the concept of
the cancer team in the cancer center has developed such that now it is virtually
the gold standard. Despite the fact that there are many excellent physicians
and surgeons in smaller towns, oncologists tend to congregate in the medical
centers, where they are part of a multidisciplinary team. Following treatment,
those patients who have come from afar are typically sent home to the care
of the referring physicians, except for the regularly scheduled follow-up visits
with the treating team. When treatment fails, the responsibility for terminal care usually falls on the referring physician. It is impractical for dying

patients to relocate to be near the cancer team that treated them, and more importantly, they generally prefer to remain in a familiar setting for the final chapter of their lives. For the cancer specialist to depend on the referring doctor at this stage is not a violation of the covenant with the patient, such as would be the case if the patient lived and died within the practice territory of the cancer physician.

Depending on the locations involved, the same problem occurs when the patient is referred into the hospice setting. In those circumstances, the patient is either back in the care of the referring physician, with whom the patient and family have a relationship, or of hospice personnel, with the primary care physician in attendance. The important thing in these circumstances is that the cancer team members see the matter through to its conclusion, that is, that they stay involved not only through communication with the medical and hospice people, but with the patient and family.

· 23 ·

Hospice Care

$\mathcal{T}$he word *hospice* refers to a concept, not necessarily a place. Both the concept and the hospice facilities, the actual place, are designed to deal only with those patients destined to die within a short and defined time frame. Given a choice, most people would probably choose to die in their own bed, so to speak, but in our busy society, there is often no one at home. The fact that 80 percent of deaths in the United States occur either in a hospice facility or in a hospital attests to our altered societal behavior. It is of academic interest only to speculate how many of the patients that do die in institutions would choose to be in more familiar surroundings if the home circumstances were different. Considering that in a substantial percentage of American homes both adults have full-time jobs and that, with a few exceptions, families do not incorporate the grandparents in the home life, it is unlikely that the situation will ever be changed. With that said, we may see changes in the hospice numbers as a result of the trend for home hospice services, in which visiting nurses provide care and comfort for the dying, even when the patient lives alone.

Regarding the hospice movement, the word itself comes from the Latin *hospis*, which means "to host"; and further, it represents a philosophy of respecting and valuing people who are dying, as well as a system of care to put that philosophy into practice. Founded in Great Britain in 1967, the movement has since taken on a major role in that society. In the United States, however, the medical profession has been slow to embrace the concept, perhaps partially for financial reasons, and probably also because of a generally paternalistic approach that existed among physicians as recently as the late 1960s. Given the circumstances of that day and time, it was counterintuitive to send a person to a place designed specifically for death since a dialogue about this then taboo subject would not have occurred. Fortunately, the

American medical profession, and especially the community of cancer physicians, has outgrown this pattern of paternalistic behavior. Exactly when the "modern approach" of disclosure and patient autonomy started is uncertain; in point of fact it has been a gradual evolution. As late as in the 1960s, physicians were still masters of avoidance and duplicity in matters pertaining to death. This was especially so with cancer patients. Hippocrates had taught physicians to comfort, but to reveal nothing of the present and the future to patients, and at least until the new approach evolved, many followed that philosophy of paternalism.

Admittedly, part of the reason was selfish—to do otherwise by a confrontation with a patient can be extremely unpleasant. Avoidance, while self-serving, was understandable. In fairness to the doctors of previous generations who withheld information, it should be pointed out that many treatments utilized today were not available, and without early diagnosis and with nothing positive to offer the patient, well-meaning physicians often sought to spare the patient from the truth, thinking that to do otherwise would be to destroy hope. The reader should consider that a 1983 Presidential Commission for the Study of Ethical Problems in Medicine said that in 1961, a cancer diagnosis was very nearly a death sentence.[1] Even though I consider that official statement to have been an overstatement, whatever caused paternalism then has largely ceased to exist, and in addition to having much more to offer in treatment, we utilize a more realistic definition of hope.

The analysis of the actual change is numerically striking. For example, in the same study cited by the presidential commission, 90 percent of doctors in 1961 said they would not tell their patients the truth about a cancer diagnosis and impending death. Another study done by the same investigators in 1978 revealed that only 3 percent of the doctors queried said they would withhold the truth. How times do change! With this change in place, the hospice movement has slowly but steadily gained acceptance, and in the last two decades, has began to flourish in the United States. A milestone of sorts was reached in 1983, when Medicare began funding hospice expenses. In 1985, hospice cared for 158,000 Americans. Since then, the numbers have increased dramatically. As a means of emphasizing these changes, of the 2.4 million people that died in 2004, 750,000 did so under hospice care.

Truth be known, the medical community has not demonstrated leadership in the promotion of the hospice movement in this country. The first hospice didn't open in the United States until 1974—seven years after the first in England; and in fact, the push in America had come largely from patients, especially cancer patients and their families.

Without question, the social climate of full disclosure had by this time changed dramatically as a result of the legal impetus for patient autonomy.

The development of the Patient Bill of Rights, powers of attorney, living wills, and the variety of informed consent protocols are but reflections of all of these social forces that had come together by that time. Actually, the development of informed consent evolved out of the law pertaining to assault and battery—that is, physicians doing things to patients without specific written permission. This is appropriately a topic of keen interest for surgeons and other interventionists. While the informed consent document does not specifically refer to a discussion of death and dying, it is an example of the change in our entire society and culture in which both physician and patient must interact and function. So while I accept the fact that the medical profession has not led the way in these societal shifts, I do believe that physicians, and especially those within the cancer world, have adapted by changing from a paternalistic and almost totally autonomous profession with virtually sacrosanct authority, to a modernized group that has subordinated its independence to group concepts such as cancer teams, multidisciplinary approaches to management, patient input, and patient autonomy. As medicine has modernized to reflect shifting social values and behavior, truthful and factual interchange, as well as an informed patient and family have become facts of life.

In sum, the hospice movement was slow to catch on in this country because, until relatively recently, the American medical profession was slow to embrace the openness with dying patients that was a necessary prerequisite to this method of aid in the process of dying. If perhaps there were financial incentives in place that mitigated the desire to embrace the hospice movement, that would certainly be an embarrassment for the profession, but it is at this point a matter of conjecture. Whatever the case, circumstances have changed and in the United States, the hospice concept is no longer viewed as a method of "dumping" dying patients, but as a means to achieve what the ancient Greeks thought of as "a tranquil death."

• *24* •

Facing Death and Dying
with the Patient

Death in itself is nothing; but we fear
To be we know not what, we know not where

—*John Dryden (1631–1700)*

It is worth noting that poets and essayists, some with wisdom, others with dramatic pontification unfounded on substance, have written much about death and dying, even though they rarely have seen it. On the other hand, the people who frequently witness death—doctors, nurses, hospice personnel, and others—rarely write about it. It follows that since death and dying are frequent companions of the cancer physician, fluency and ease of conversation with the relevant dialogue are essential. With that said, my initial advice to future oncologists is to critically look within and attempt to understand the most personal of their own feelings that relate to the variety of relevant issues. And those already on the pathway to this subspecialty should forgo leadership in these matters until they have undergone self-analysis and contemplation of their own beliefs and attitudes about death-related issues.

Self-knowledge is essential before discussing death and dying with a patient. How can a dying strategy that fits a patient and family be promoted absent the physician's clear vision on such matters as suicide, generally; physician-assisted suicide, specifically; physician assisted death, that is, terminal sedation; and the role of hospice care in the dying process. It should always be remembered that during the final approach to death, the oncologist is the go-to person for patient and family in a variety of matters. While much of what concerns them can and will be handled by the supporting team, many of the questions asked are well within the purview of a mature oncologist, and the patient and family should get the sense that their physician is involved and overseeing almost everything that's happening.

Granted, the dilemmas associated with dying have been somewhat mitigated in modern times by the employment of living wills and other legal documents in which specific instructions about limitations of care are given. It's surprising, however, how few patients die with a living will in place, and even when they do, there can be many unresolved issues. An alternative to the living will is the health care power of attorney that is less complicated, which entrusts certain designees with authority to make decisions, presumably based on predeath discussions with the patient. While this may have the advantage of legal simplicity, and while it may fit certain trusted domestic and family relationships, such a document introduces the vulnerabilities resulting from family dysfunction in which "loved ones" choose to follow the rapacious instincts of estate benefactors. Even when legal documents accomplish their intended purpose in directing the medical team during the final stages of a life with specific dos and don'ts, and even when the family is functional and cooperative, the physician must deal with many human components while helping patient and family with death.

While there usually are multiple medical persons in contact with a cancer patient, fragmented discussions about death should be avoided. The alpha oncologist or that member of the cancer team closest to the patient and family ought to be the person to conduct any specific death and dying discussion. There is an understandable tendency among oncologists to avoid pessimistic information with patients and their families. Essentially, they prefer to discuss possibilities of remission or disease control rather than impending death. Nevertheless, it is essential that the appropriate people handle the issues that pertain to the final chapter of life.

By and large, in our contemporary society, the standard is to avoid the paternalism that leads doctors to keep the truth from patients about impending death. To paraphrase Nuland again, the worst form of paternalism is the withholding of information because of the fear that the patient might use it to make a wrong decision.[1] Unless we know early on that we might die, or that we are actually dying, how are we able to reconcile our lives and our relationships and rectify certain mistakes? How is all of this possible without an honest and forthright discussion with one's physician? With a well-crafted discussion, there often follows an element of surrender to the reality of death, understandably sometimes accompanied by anxiety, but usually without terror. More often, the surrender is followed by acceptance and a sense of calm—in the vernacular of the hospice philosophy, a tranquil comfort, rather than turbulence and rampant fear of the unknown. To paraphrase Kathleen Dowling Singh, this passage from realization to acceptance is essential to the willingness of a patient to cease trying to hold at bay the reality of their mortality.[2]

I vividly recall my mother's death. A week or so before she actually died, she had been put on a respirator, but except for being mildly sedated, was awake. Prevented by the respirator from talking, she wrote prolific notes to me about my responsibilities to the family. She even amended her will while on the respirator (imagine lawyers in the ICU), making special arrangements for the care of a family member that she was particularly concerned about. She was clear and determined to take care of business, and visited individually with each close member of the family for reasons that surely related in her mind to closure. All of this started the day after she had written a note to me—her son the doctor—pointedly asking if she was going to die. When I answered this very painful question with a "probably" (she did not have cancer, and there was still some uncertainty), she nodded and made it clear to me that she was ready. I thought later how she would have been cheated by avoidance of the truth at that specific moment. Knowing my mother, I had anticipated the question, and it was logical that it would be directed to me; and while the temptation to reassure her with unrealistic words was strong, I knew that I must respond truthfully. Not to do so, while initially protective, would have robbed her of the opportunity to accept and surrender. She didn't give up, but instead surrendered to the inevitability of death, and in doing so, was able to reaffirm relationships with loved ones and also to bring closure to various matters of importance. As the end drew near, she was sedated and probably in no pain. In many ways, it was a good and tranquil death.

The degree of fear of death varies between individuals. For some, the whole notion is terrifying and uncertain, while for others it is an anticipated journey to another place—perhaps a better place where reunion with love ones will occur. When there is fear and trepidation, Singh believes that much of it relates to the loss of control and an entrance into the unknown. Perhaps the viewing of death as the end of one's existence and the fear of subsequent nothingness and oblivion are also part of the equation. I have watched a number of patients enter and go through the final glide path to death, and I am impressed with several facts: Younger people have the hardest time with death, perhaps because of the anger and sense of having been cheated out of potential accomplishments; young mothers revert to very basic maternal concerns for their children, and in some there is a sense of guilt for deserting them; the elderly do best with the knowledge of impending death, often because of a long anticipation of the final exit, or perhaps out of a sense of relief from loneliness, or because they are happy to abandon suffering and disability.

The tranquility of the elderly perhaps comes from having had the opportunity to resolve such life challenges as intimacy and achievement. Not infrequently, it is the elderly patient who is worried about their surviving loved ones, rather than the reverse. On a number of occasions, I have witnessed such dying patients trying to comfort those around them.

Patients with a strong spiritual foundation—belief in life after death, heaven, the existence of God—are confident in the fact that the totality of their goodness will be rewarded by entry into *that place*. Such patients more often die a tranquil death. It is worth noting that while most believers feel that one is judged on the totality of life, Roman Catholic doctrine goes one step further and teaches that it is also important to die in "the state of grace"—a level that is guaranteed by receiving the last rites of the church (Extreme Unction). Entrance into heaven is thereby assured.

Other religious people view life on earth merely as a trial in which one pays dues for entrance into a better life. One of my favorite relatives, a different great-uncle than the one I mentioned at the outset of this book, said to me just before he died that no one should grieve for him. The only concern should be for those that loved him and who would feel the loneliness that resulted from his absence. He had been blessed with a long life that had been extraordinary and fulfilling, and he genuinely looked forward to even better things ahead. At the time, my thought was that it was wonderful to leave life's stage with a spiritual smile.

SPECIFICS OF THE ACTUAL
DEATH AND DYING DISCUSSION

A modified death and dying discussion—hypothetical and not so peppered with specific details—can occur during the initial stage of physician-patient contact, depending on circumstances and the patient's needs. If, for instance, the patient is failing to realistically deal with a newly diagnosed cancer—for example trying to put off the treatment, or considering alternative methods of treatment—it is essential that there be a discussion that includes almost certain death if standard therapy is not employed. In other patients in whom there is optimism for cure and in whom the specific treatment is being planned, the patient might poses the question, "What if the treatment fails . . . then what?" I have generally avoided an in-depth discussion based on the hypothetical "what if," since it can stimulate much anxiety; however, in such a circumstance, some overview is unavoidable. Often we have second and even third lines of defense after the primary therapy fails, but in each tier there is a lessened chance of cure.

The "real" as opposed to the "modified" discussion is the main thrust of this section. There is no specific time for the obligatory death and dying discussion, as long as it is not during the final glide path to the end. Generally speaking, it should take place at some earlier point of the cancer's progression, after the inevitability of death is clear. When is best depends on a number of circumstances. In those patients, however, in whom therapy has failed and the battle is lost, or in whom the situation is deemed hopeless from the outset, the cancer physician's role is critical early on and becomes more so as death approaches. For the lead oncologist not to accept this responsibility or not to stay involved and available until the end is tantamount to abandonment.

First and foremost, I believe that it is counterproductive and perhaps even wrong to shade the truth from most patients. Simply put, patients should know they are facing death. I have devoted considerable thought to this issue during my professional life, and my feelings have vacillated from the paternalistic protection of patient ignorance early in my career to my current belief in full disclosure. I agree with Nuland that the most comfortless and solitary way to die is when the knowledge of death's certainty is withheld. Unless we are aware that we are dying and to some extent know the conditions of our death, we are unable to share final consummation with those who love us. Without this, no matter their presence at the time of death, we remain unattended and isolated.

During the actual discussion, patients frequently ask how long they have to live. Dealing with this question is tricky; therefore, oncologists instinctively avoid answering it. Studies have shown that in those instances in which physicians predicted a specific time until death, only 20 percent did so with reasonable accuracy.[3] The data suggest that they tend to overestimate the predictive time by a multiple of 5. The fact remains, however, that not being good at estimating the unpredictable is not justification for avoiding the discussion. In my experience, patients readily accept a general time frame for how long they have left to live. I have always responded to the question by saying that "it's impossible to be too specific, but probably a matter of months, rather than years," or something to that effect. Committing to a very general time frame as opposed to merely saying it's unpredictable allows the patient to plan better. I have had patients live with cancers that have slowed dramatically—to virtual dormancy—so as to exceed the predicted time of life by years. Such an event is the exception, however, and most patterns of cancer death are steadily downhill.

In the beginning of the journey to death, the oncologist's role is one of guidance and leadership, and the honesty of a carefully chosen vocabulary that is retrieved from the physician's philosophy about what lies ahead is usually very helpful to the patient. There are few things in medicine more abhorrent than telling a patient and a family that the battle with cancer has been lost, or even that it is hopeless before the battle begins. It is undoubtedly better that the discussion only be undertaken by the few who know the natural history of the offending disease and the mechanics of terminal events, who know all of the options available, and who have the self-confidence to make direct eye contact with patient and family and to speak in understandable and definitive lingo—all the while being compassionate, tender, and honest. For this zone of communication to be entered by a physician who is squeamish, self-conscious, and not grounded in the full knowledge of the topic is usually fraught with problems of patient confidence and unresolved fears, perpetuated ignorance, and a much more turbulent journey to the end. The physician must represent a pillar of reliability and steadiness at this very emotional juncture, and must demonstrate a take-charge attitude that inspires the confidence that the final stages of life will be well orchestrated.

The death and dying discussion should be the responsibility of the lead oncologist whenever possible—or the oncologist on the team who has the closest relationship with patient and family. I have always welcomed this responsibility in patients to whom I am close, because it is clear to me what works best in helping people deal with impending death. That's not to say that others with whom I have worked are not just as able in their own right, and many of them probably feel the same way about their own capabilities. This is an example of what I mean about the importance of the physician's self-confidence.

As part of the death and dying discussion—no matter when held—the patient's own philosophy about death should be seriously considered and incorporated. This is easier said than done, and what ideally should be a dialogue can end up being a monologue in which the doctor does all the talking. The ease and the communicative competence of the physician are important to the unfolding of this process. Importantly, the patient should feel free to reject recommendations without fear of being devalued as a patient. The whole conversation may seem like tedious dwelling on the negative, but in my experience, just the opposite is true; and surprisingly, many patients have already considered many of the issues. Some patients want empathetic discussions about outcomes and possibilities, no matter how ominous they might be. Not infrequently, such a patient asks for a description of what their terminal time will be like. How does this cancer kill—how will I die? Will there be much pain? Will I have trouble breathing and swallowing? Will I undergo the indignity of incontinence? Can I be with my family at the time of death? Will I stink as the cancer grows? Can I die at home? Can I be in a hospice or will I have to stay in a hospital? It is a contradiction of our times that, when asked, a large percentage of people say they would prefer to die at home, unattached to machines, and in the bosom of familiar surroundings and people; yet in the United States, such is not what really happens the majority of the time. Except for those who die unexpectedly, 80 percent of deaths in America now occur either in hospitals or hospice facilities. There are a number of sociologic factors that enter into this.

I mentioned above a question not infrequently asked by patients, about whether they will have a foul odor as their cancer progresses. I refer to this to make the specific point that an in-depth death-and-dying dialogue can be a graphic experience. It is difficult to teach young doctors how to regulate this discussion. In practical fact, the patient most often dictates the desired degree of explicitness. Whatever that level of specificity, the most believable discussion is almost always the honest one. For instance, I mentioned odors in the preceding paragraph; this is no small consideration to the person destined to die from one of the malignancies that have external exposure—skin; rectum; breast; colostomy sites; aero-digestive sites such as tongue, sinuses, and so on. As a result of outgrowing their own blood supply, these cancers become necrotic, superficially infected, and malodorous. It's difficult for a physician, no matter how linguistically capable, to circumvent or minimize the patient's concern for a repugnant source of decay, in which vanity, dignity, and self-loathing are part of the equation. So when asked, to be other than honest is to risk one's overall credibility with the patient and family.

On a number of occasions, I have witnessed prolonged cancer deaths that have been associated with the worst of these factors, and even when the patient is terminally sedated, the family often avoids entering the mephitic atmosphere of the room. Often, family members are relieved and even somewhat happy when the end finally comes. Not surprisingly, many of those who experience such emotions feel guilty.

Toward the end, some cancers grow at a dramatic pace, but when they don't encroach on vital structures, the patient can linger, even when deprived of sustenance. Simultaneously, a cancer uses the body's energy stores, and the resultant malnutrition creates a cascade of events. Normally, the body counters starvation by using its fat stores, but in rampant cancer, protein is utilized at the expense of organ function and muscle mass. The wasted appearance and sallow color of cancer cachexia can be ugly as well as unforgettable, and when this state is combined with foul odors, terminal time is better shortened, rather than prolonged. Physician-author Sherwin Nuland achieves the full power of descriptive metaphor in his wonderfully written book *How We Die* by describing rampant cancer as pursuing a continuous, uninhibited, circumferential expedition of destructiveness, with its cells behaving like members of a barbarian horde run amok; and in which, in the end, there is no victory for the cancer—when it kills its victim, it kills itself.[4]

DEATH—NATURE'S FINAL DEBT

If I must die, I will encounter darkness as a bride,
and hug it in my arms.

William Shakespeare (1564–1616)

It was with no slight consideration that I have on several occasions in this writing used the phrase, a *journey to death*. The passage is discussed in two treatises from the Middle Ages known as *Ars Moriendi* ("The Art of Dying").[5] These works created a cartographic outline of the psycho-spiritual transformations of the dying process. In effect, dying people were considered to be moving by pilgrimage into a spiritual dimension. That depiction of death, however, reflected the mind-set of that bygone era, and whatever applicability there is today is left for esoteric lamentations.

Since that period, technological advancements have substantially altered the dynamics of death. Most people who avoid sudden death and who go on to succumb to a chronic illness such as cancer die in an altered state of twilight or even unconsciousness that has been induced by drugs. In times of yore, the hour of death was a time of spiritual sanctity and last communion with those left behind. In most situations today, however, drugs have altered that state. Essentially, important end of life matters—goodbyes and other matters of reconciliation—must precede what I refer to as the final glide path to death.

It should be pointed out, however, that the principles at the core of the hospice concept have fostered a renewed emphasis on redefining the quality of death so as to encourage exodus with a minimum of chemical influence but a maximum of counseling. Kathleen Dowling Singh refers to death as an occasion of profound spiritual significance, and in her reference to the nearing death experience, refers to the great mystery at the edge of life and death.[6] In reading her book, *The Grace of Dying*, I was initially skeptical of its practical applicability; however, the more I read, the more intuitive I found the reasoning of the author. Ironically, we spend our entire adult life conceding the inevitability of death, only to push back when we finally face it; and much of the death counseling advocated by Singh is designed to overcome what she refers to as the hardwired instinct of self-preservation.

It is certainly a mystery to me whether death comes in an instant or, as some believe, in a continuum of spiritual transformation and gradual withdrawal. Repeatedly, certain authors refer to the "nearing death experience" and in those patients who are unencumbered by drugs, I am intrigued by the claim that a substantial percentage of them, perhaps 10 percent or more, report vivid visions of deceased love ones in the hour that immediately precede death. As a concrete-thinking surgeon, I have always equated the moment of death with the cessation of brain and cardiovascular activities on the various monitors. In Singh's book, she writes that she has on many occasions experienced a sense of atmospheric change at the moment of death, or a "woosh," as she says. Importantly, this is not an observation unique to that author's experience. Such transcendental claims may be rooted in the recognized but little understood bioenergy fields that surround and interpenetrate the interstices of the body.

Since I lack the depth of knowledge to refute the notion of a passage or transition over time, I prefer to stick with my belief that death is an abrupt phenomenon; however, I see no reason why the two unproven hypotheses cannot coexist. In reflecting back, I must say that I have on several occasions experienced what Singh referred to when I have felt a palpable change in the atmosphere at the time of a patient's death. Most dramatic in my memory is when my mother died, and at the very second that I watched the monitors flatline, I felt this odd sensation like something leaving the room. My sister—unprompted by me, confessed to experiencing the same sensation. Could that be the "woosh" that Singh has written about? I have spoken to a number of other people, including physicians who have had similar experiences. Much research is being done on bioelectrical energy fields associated with life, and this, including the "woosh," provides fodder for discussion in the halls of neurobiology. At a minimum, and on a practical level, it should give some pause each time a person writes on a legal form the actual time of death—does that represent precision or not?

Epilogue

$\mathcal{T}$o say that we are entering times that are sociologically, medically, ethically, and philosophically challenging is inaccurate because that would suggest something new, when in fact, dramatic changes have been ongoing for some time. To speculate on a specific time frame is virtually impossible, but I suspect insidious change has been beneath our radar screen for quiet a while. To a large extent, what we are experiencing is the dramatization of issues and a changing paradigm that are driven by rapidly increasing information being shared throughout the world. There are so many unanswered and perhaps unanswerable questions before us, and as is appropriate, many will be left for future generation to deal with. After all, they are the ones who will have to live with the consequences of their answers and decisions.

What I have attempted to do in this writing is to influence the future perception of the medical profession as being best functioning in a state of symbiosis with the nonmedical world. At the heart of my search is the implication that I really do feel that the two are different and apart, but that their coexistence is not only possible but workable. This is not an elitist notion that attempts to rank the profession above any other; that would imply a competitiveness that truly does not exist. Instead, I think of physicians as public servants who are willing to take on critical responsibilities that other people would not even consider, and, by virtue of their willingness to accept this intensity of lifestyle and responsibilities, ought to be thought of differently than other public servants. I have sought to promote a traditional medical system within a changing social framework by emphasizing certain basic values that I believe have the strength to survive the most dramatic social changes. Without question, physicians must adapt and change, and as a result of doing so, there will be discomfort among them. However, as the world around us changes, the one thing that physicians must retain is a sense of self-worth that is based on an altruistic model. Despite the many absurd bureaucratic demons constantly nibbling at our core, and despite the forces that seek to make us the same as other public servants, our mission—the improvement of the human condition—should be valued and protected. For the profession to deal with these changes and forces by compromising ethical and educational standards—by abandoning those principles that have connected us to a moral center—is to invite a certain slide into further irrelevance. If we allow this to happen, future generations will longingly look back and think how good American medicine once was.

In doing the research necessary to write this book, I interviewed a number of former cancer patients, most of whom I had treated, but some others from other venues—prostate gland, lung, breast, and other malignancies. My discussions were extraordinarily informative, and they served to help me synthesize and formulate much of what I have included in this text. Significantly, I heard consistent themes—over and over—about fear, chronic post-treatment anxiety, emotional dependence on their physicians, the desperate need to trust, and a desire to follow real leadership by those in whom they had placed their trust. The need to idealize the medical profession, while somewhat altered through the cataract of modern society, is still more than fantasy—it's real. Much more came out of these interviews than I have specifically mentioned. Hopefully, I have at least peripherally touched on much that will provide a stimulus for reflection and discussion.

By teaching one almost always learns. So it is with writing, especially when the subject is sociologically so relevant. I mentioned earlier that while I was planning this book I had no idea how involved I would become in the whole topic of whether physicians ought to ever be killers as well as healers, that is, should they ever be involved with euthanasia and physician-assisted suicide. For me it was not enough to research the topic, and until I attempted to articulate my beliefs on paper, my philosophy was ambivalent. Not so now! This experience has convinced me that the Slippery Slope theory is real, and physicians should stand squarely against participation, no matter how relentless the social forces. In the long term, no matter the constraints, evil in the name of expedience will usurp the expectation of good. To risk such a descent into immorality is not and will never be justified. Importantly, we must not hesitate or equivocate about getting involved in the social debate that will forge ahead—with us, or without us. In researching this topic, I discussed the state laws regarding physician-assisted suicide with several medical leaders of several of the states that allow this. In each, they were unaware of the details, but each was quick to say they could never participate in such an act. Such passivity does not represent what I believe our proactive role in this debate ought to be. By virtue of this book, our medical leadership should consider picking up the flag that I have staked.

As we search for professional redemption and preservation, my advocacy for reliance on the ethics and values of our forefathers is actually a by-product of my original intent, which was to influence aspirants in the world of oncology. As the book developed, however, the two themes blended together. Using cancer as a focal point for the book serves a dual purpose: first, the advocacy of those basic values that should be common to all physicians; and second, making the case that more than any other endeavor in medicine, caring for cancer patients involves an extended commitment that, while enormously gratifying, demands a high emotional price. The price to which I refer is not necessarily a burden—that is a subjective and relative label; however, the commitment is real and it is consuming. Essentially, the cancer specialist cannot bounce in and out of patients' lives, and that fact more than any other separates us from our counterparts in the noncancer world.

I have declared that patients are never quite the same emotionally after undergoing *the cancer experience*. In a sense, cancer physicians share that transformation as a result of caring for this very needy population. When the symphony of interacting forces and parts between physician and patient is functional, the emotional rewards for both are sublime.

Roy B. Sessions, MD, FACS
Charleston, South Carolina

Notes

CHAPTER 1

1. By "academic physician" I mean to include the full-time academicians based in medical centers, the many part-time academicians, and also those physicians in private practice who fill an important role by teaching clinical medicine to those in training.

2. Thomas Jefferson, Letter to John Adams, October 28, 1813, in *The Life and Selected Writings of Jefferson*, ed. Adrienne Kock and William Peden (New York: Random House, 1944), 632.

CHAPTER 2

1. *Psyche* can be defined as the psychological structure of a person, especially as a motivating force.

2. Bertrand Russell, *The Autobiography of Bertrand Russell* (New York: Routledge, 2000).

3. Winston Churchill, *Their Finest Hours* (Boston: Houghton, Mifflin, 1999), 360.

CHAPTER 3

1. Thomas Smith, "Cancer Care: A Microcosm of the Problems Facing All of Health Care," *Annuals of Internal Medicine* 150, no. 8 (2009): 576.

CHAPTER 4

1. Eric J. Cassell, *Doctoring: The Nature of Primary Care Medicine* (New York: Oxford University Press, 1997).

2. John Diamond, *Because Cowards Get Cancer Too* (New York: Times Books 1998), x.

3. Sidney Winawer on the cover of Jimmie Holland and Sheldon Lewis, *The Human Side of Cancer: Living with Hope, Coping with Uncertainty* (New York: HarperCollins, 1999).

4. Psycho-oncology is a relatively new psychiatric subspecialty that began in the mid-1970s and deals with the psychological issues relating to cancer.

CHAPTER 5

1. Jerome Groopman, *The Anatomy of Hope* (New York: Random House, 2005).

2. Groopman, *Anatomy of Hope*, xiv.

3. Jimmie Holland, and Sheldon Lewis, *The Human Side of Cancer* (HarperCollins, 1999), 13–25.

4. Walter Scott, Quote from *The New Dictionary of Thoughts*, ed. Tryon Edwards, rev. and enl. by C. N. Catrevas, Jonathan Edwards, and Ralph Emerson Browns (New York: Standard Book Company, 1961), 279.

5. Groopman, *Anatomy of Hope*, 39.

6. Kathleen Dowling Singh, *The Grace in Dying* (New York: HarperCollins, 1998), 13.

7. Peter Ubel, "Cancer Care: A Microcosm of the Problems Facing All of Health Care," *Annuals of Internal Medicine* 150, no. 8 (2009): 573.

8. The last rites, or extreme unction, is a Roman Catholic sacrament in which the dying person is anointed with oil while prayers are recited by a priest.

9. Lucius Annaeus Seneca (also known as Seneca the Younger) was a Roman Stoic philosopher, statesman, dramatist, and humorist. As a Roman senator he was ordered by Caesar to commit suicide. (4 BC–AD 65).

10. Sherwin B. Nuland, *How We Die: Reflections on Life's Final Chapter* (New York: Vintage Books, 1995), 260.

11. Singh, *The Grace in Dying*, 270.

12. Centers for Disease Control and Prevention, Cancer, in press.

13. President's Cancer Panel, *NCI Annual Report, 2004–2005* (Washington, DC: National Cancer Institute), Part 1, 1.

14. U.S. Census Bureau, "Current Population Report" (Washington, DC: U.S. Census Bureau, 1993), 25–1104.

15. B. K. Edwards, H. L. Howe, L. A. Ries, M. H. Thun, H. M. Rosenberg, R. Yancik, P. A. Wingo, A. Jermal, and E. G. Feigal, *Annual Report to the Nation on the Status of Cancer 1973–1999*, *Cancer* 94, no. 10 (2002): 2766–92.

16. Medicare Payment Advisory Commission, "Medicare Payments for Outpatient Drugs under Part B," in *Report to the Congress: Variation and Innovation in Medicare*, June 2005 (accessed on 17 March 2009 at http://www.medpac.gov/publications%5Ccongressional_reports%5CJune03_Ch9.pdf).

17. F. J. Emanuel, Y. Young-Xu, N. G. Levinsky, G. Gazelle, O. Saynina, and A. S. Ash, "Chemotherapy Use among Medicare Beneficiaries at the End of Life," *Ann Inter Med.* 138 (2003): 639–43 [PMID: 12693886].

18. C. C. Eagle, B. A. Neville, M. B. Landrum, J. Ayanian, S. D. Block, and J. C. Weeks, "Trends in the Aggressiveness of Cancer Care Near the End of Life," *J Clin Oncol* 22 (2004): 315–21 [PMID: 14722041].

19. Jennifer Fisher Wilson, "Editorial on Cancer Care: A Microcosm of the Problems Facing All of Health Care," *Annals of Int Medicine* 150, no. 8 (2009): 573.

20. President's Cancer Panel, *NCI Annual Report, 2004–2005*.

CHAPTER 6

1. I borrow the phrase "Cancer Olympics" from Marion Morra and Eve Potts, *Choices* (New York: Avon Books, 1994).

CHAPTER 7

1. Thomas Jefferson quoted in Sherwin B. Nuland, *How We Die: Reflections on Life's Final Chapter* (New York: Vintage Books, 1995).

2. A deist is a person who believes the Creator does not interfere in human affairs.

3. Stephen E. Ambrose, *Undaunted Courage* (New York: Simon & Schuster 1996), chap. 30.

4. Quoted in Nuland, *How We Die*, 44.

5. Edmund D. Pellegrino, "The John Conley Lecture," delivered to the Annual Meeting of the American Academy of Otolaryngology / Head and Neck Surgery, San Diego, CA, September 8, 1990.

CHAPTER 8

1. Edmund D. Pellegrino, "The John Conley Lecture," delivered to the Annual Meeting of the American Academy of Otolaryngology / Head and Neck Surgery, San Diego, CA September 8, 1990.

2. Pellegrino, "The John Conley Lecture."

CHAPTER 9

1. A pessary is a device worn in the vagina to support the uterus, but was used by ancients to induce abortion.

2. *Roe v. Wade*, 410 U.S. 113 (1973).

3. E. J. Furton, P. Cataldo, and O. Andmoraczewski, eds., *Catholic Health Care Ethics: A Manual for Practitioners*, 2nd ed. (Philadelphia, PA: National Catholic Bioethics Center, 2009), 23.

4. John Donne, quoted in preface of Ernest Hemingway, *For Whom the Bell Tolls* (New York: P. F. Collier and Son, 1940).

CHAPTER 10

1. Sherwin B. Nuland, *How We Die: Reflections on Life's Final Chapter* (New York: Vintage Books, 1995), 8.

2. Margaret Pabst Battin, *Ending Life: Ethics and the Way We Die* (New York: Oxford University Press, 2005), 37.

3. Michael Burleigh, *Death and Deliverance: "Euthanasia" in Germany 1900–1945* (Cambridge: Cambridge University Press, 1995), chap. 1.

4. Euripides as quoted in *Bartlett's Familiar Quotations*, 15th ed. (New York: Little, Brown), 77.

5. Neal Bascomb, *Hunting Eichmann: How a Band of Survivors and a Young Spy Agency Chased Down the World's Most Notorious Nazi* (New York: Houghton Mifflin Harcourt, 2009).

6. Burleigh, *Death and Deliverance*, 27.

7. Burleigh, *Death and Deliverance*, 15.

8. Burleigh, *Death and Deliverance*, 24.

9. Burleigh, *Death and Deliverance*, 20.

10. Gerald Dworkin, R. Frey, and Sissela Bok, *Euthanasia and Physician-Assisted Suicide: For and Against* (Cambridge: Cambridge University Press 1998), 125.

11. "Law Sought in China on Euthanasia," *Boston Globe*, March 15, 1996, 7.

12. Tim Johnson, "Columbia High Court Approves Mercy Killing," *Boston Globe*, May 22, 1997, 7.

13. Debora Ball, and Julia Mengewein, "Assisted Suicide Pioneer Stirs Legal Backlash," *Wall Street Journal*, February 6–7, 2010.

14. Battin, *Ending Life*, 57.

15. Aldous Huxley, *Brave New World* (Garden City, NY: Doubleday).

16. Battin, *Ending Life*, 52.

17. P. Admiral, "Euthanasia in a General Hospital" (paper read at the Eighth World Congress of the International Federation of Right to Die Societies, Maastricht, The Netherlands, June 1990).

18. Sissela Bok, "Euthanasia" in *Euthanasia and Physician Assisted Suicide*, G. Dworkin, R. Frey, and S. Bok (Cambridge University Press, 1998), 123–24.

19. Leon Kass, *Life, Liberty, and the Defense of Dignity* (New York: Encounter Books, 2002), 2078.

20. Bok, "Euthanasia," 124.

21. Battin, *Ending Life.*

22. This information regarding various state legislative attempts to legalize euthanasia and/or physician assisted suicide was gathered by the International Task Force on Euthanasia and Assisted Suicide, P.O. Box 760, Steubenville, OH, 43952.

23. Quoted in Dworkin, Frey, and Bok, *Euthanasia and Physician-Assisted Suicide*, 47.

24. Battin, *Ending Life*, 26.

25. Niccolo Machiavelli, *The Prince* (New York: Oxford University Press, 2008), 53.

26. C. L. Sprung, "Changing Attitudes and Practices in Forgoing Life Sustaining Treatments," *JAMA* 263 (1990): 2213.

27. T. Pendergast, and J. M. Luce, "Increasing Incidence of Withholding and Withdrawal of Life Support from the Critically Ill," *Am Journal of Respiratory and Critical Care Medicine* 155 (1): 1–2.

28. S. Miles, and C. Gomez, *Protocols for Elective Use of Life-Sustaining Treatments* (New York: Springer-Verlag, 1988).

CHAPTER 11

1. V. Gajalakshmim, and R. Peto, "Suicide Rates in Rural Tamil Nadu, South India: Verbal Autopsy of 39,000 Deaths in 1997–98," *Int. J. Epidemiol* 36 (2007): 203–7.

2. M. R. Philips, X. Li, and Y. Zhang, "Suicide Rates in China, 1995–99," *Lancet* 359 (2002): 835–40.

3. Sidney Bloch, and Stephen Green, eds., *Psychiatric Ethics*, 4th ed. (New York: Oxford University Press, 2009), 229.

4. World Health Organization, *World Report on Violence and Health* (Geneva, Switzerland: World Health Organization, 2002); World Health Organization, *World Health Statistics* (Geneva, Switzerland: World Health Organization, 1989).

5. F. Levi, C. Lavecchia, F. Lucchini, et al., "Trends in Mortality from Suicide, 1965–99," *Acta Psychiatr Scand.* 108, no. 5 (November 2003): 341–49.

6. J. T. Cavanaugh, A. Carson, M. Sharpe, and S. Lawrie, "Psychological Autopsy Studies of Suicide: A Systematic Review," *Psychol Med* 33 (2003): 395–403.

7. F. Goodwin, and K. Jamison, *Manic-Depressive: Bipolar Disorders and Recurrent Depression*, 2nd ed. (New York: Oxford University Press, 2007).

8. S. Fazel, J. Cartwright, A. Nott-Norman, and K. Hawton, "Suicide in Prisoners: A Systematic Review of Risk Factors," *J Clin Psychiatry* 69 (2008): 1721–31; M. King, J. Semlyen, S. Seetai, et al., "A Systematic Review of Mental Disorder, Suicide,

and Deliberate Self-Harm in Lesbian, Gay, and Bisexual People," *BMC Psychiatry* 8 (August 18, 2008): 70.

9. Michal Harwood, et al., "Life Problems and Physical Illness as Risk Factors for Suicide in Older People: A Descriptive Case-Control Study," *Psychological Medicine* 36, no. 9 (September 2006): 1265–74.

10. D. Carney, and S. Horton-Deutsh, "Suicide Over 60: The San Diego Study," *J Am Geriatr Soc.* 42, no. 2 (February 1994): 174–80; M. Waern, E. Rubenowitz, et al., "Burden of Illness and Suicide in Elderly People: A Case-Control Study," *British Medical Journal* 324 (June 8, 2002): 1355–57.

11. Harwood, Hawton, et al., "Life Problems and Physical Illness as Risk Factors for Suicide."

12. M. Llorente, M. Burke, C. Gregory, et al., "Prostate Cancer: A Significant Risk Factor for Late-Life Suicide," *Am J. Geriatr Psychiatry* 13, no. 3 (2005): 195–201.

13. M. Miller, H. Mogun, D. Azreal, et al., "Cancer and the Risk of Suicide in Older Americans," *J Clin Oncol* 26, no. 29 (2008): 4720–24.

14. W. Kendal, "Suicide and Cancer: A Gender-Comparative Study," *Ann Oncol* 18 (2007): 381–87; N. Dormer, K. McCaul, and L. Kristjanson, "Risk of Suicide in Cancer Patients in Western Australia, 1981–2002," *Med J Aust* 88, no. 3 (2008): 140–43.

15. R. Howard, P. Inskip, and L. Travis, "Suicide after Childhood Cancer," *J Clin Oncol* 25 (2009): 731.

16. C. Recklitis, R. Lockwood, M. Rothwell, et al., "Suicidal Ideation and Attempts in Adult Survivors of Childhood Cancer," *J Clin Oncol* 24, no. 24 (2006): 3852–57.

17. G. Li, "The Interaction Effect of Bereavement and Sex on the Risk of Suicide in the Elderly: An Historic Cohort Study," *Social Science and Medicine* 40 (1995): 825–28.

18. W. Pirl, and A. Roth, "A Diagnosis and Treatment of Depression in Cancer Patients," *Oncology* 13, no. 9 (1999): 1293–1301.

19. D. Rasic, S. Belik, J. Bolton, et al., "Cancer, Mental Disorders, Suicidal Ideations, and Attempts in a Large Community Sample," *Psycho-Oncology* 17 (2008): 660–67.

20. M. Resnick, "Protecting Adolescents from Harm: Findings from the National Longitudinal Study on Adolescent Health," *JAMA* 278, no. 10 (September 1997): 823–32.

21. Zenon of Citium (c. 334–c. 262 BC) was a Greek philosopher who allegedly founded the school of philosophy of stoicism.

CHAPTER 14

1. The "Big C" is a colloquialism that comes from a not to distant time when the word *cancer* carried a shameful stigma and there was an effort to avoid using it.

CHAPTER 16

1. George Eliot, *Middlemarch* (London: Blackwood and Sons, 1874).

CHAPTER 18

1. Quoted in *Bartlett's Famous Quotations*, 15th ed. (New York: Little, Brown, 1980), 703.

2. The phrase "the balm of adulation" is borrowed from the writings of contemporary journalist and columnist George Will.

3. Quoted in *Bartlett's Famous Quotations* 15th ed. (New York: Little, Brown, 1980), 907.

CHAPTER 20

1. Translational research is a way of conducting scientific research to make the results applicable to the population under study.

2. President's Cancer Panel, "NCI Annual Report," 2004–2005, Part 1, 1.

3. Jeffrey Kluger, "How Faith Can Heal," *Time*, February 23, 2009.

4. See Lucius Annaeus Seneca, Excerpts from Letter 70 in the series of Letters to Lucilius, in *The Stoic Philosophy of Seneca*, ed. and trans. Moses Hadas (New York: W. W. Norton, 1958).

5. Marion Morra and Eve Potts, *Choices* (Avon Books, 1994), 742.

CHAPTER 21

1. Peter Ubel, "Cancer Care: A Microcosm of the Problems Facing All of Health Care," *Annuals of Internal Medicine* 150, no. 8 (2009): 573.

CHAPTER 22

1. The wake is a medieval custom, not necessarily of Roman Catholic creation, but one that is perpetuated in contemporary Catholic funeral ritual, in which a watch or vigil over the body of the deceased is held before burial. In times prior to the rapidity of modern transportation, a period of days or more were allotted for family members

and friends to travel from afar to attend the funeral procession. During that time, the body of the deceased is displayed around the clock in the funeral parlor, usually with a family member in attendance. By contrast, traditional Judaism requires a burial shortly after death, and the ritual equivalent to the wake is known in Hebrew as the shivah—a period of mourning in which friends and family visit the survivors of the deceased in a social venue, without the deceased. The verb is utilized in the expression "to sit shivah."

CHAPTER 23

1. President's Commission for the Study of Ethical Problems in Medicine and Biomedical and Behavioral Research, *Deciding to Forego Life-Sustaining Treatment* (Washington, DC: U.S. Government Printing Office,1983), 52–53.

CHAPTER 24

1. Sherwin Nuland, *How We Die: Reflections on Life's Final Chapter* (New York: Vintage Books, 1995), 252.
2. Kathleen Dowling Singh, *The Grace in Dying* (HarperCollins, 1998).
3. N. Christakis, and E. Lamont, "Extent and Determinations of Error in Doctors Prognosis in Terminally Ill Patients," *British Med Journal* 320 (February 19, 2000): 469–73.
4. Nuland, *How We Die*, 10.
5. According to Wikipedia: "The *Ars moriendi* ('The Art of Dying') are two related Latin texts dating from about 1415 and 1450 which offer advice on the protocols and procedures of a good death, explaining how to 'die well' according to Christian precepts of the late Middle Ages." Wikipedia http://en.wikipedia.org/wiki/Ars_moriendi
6. Singh, *The Grace of Dying*, 269–79.

Bibliography

Ambrose, Stephen E. *Undaunted Courage*. New York: Simon & Schuster, 1996.

Admiral, P, *Euthanasia in a General Hospital*. Paper read at the 8th World Congress of the International Federation of Right to Die Societies, Maastricht, The Netherlands, June 1990.

Ball, Debra, and Julie Mengewein. "Assisted Suicide Pioneer Stirs Legal Backlash." *Wall Street Journal*, February 6–7, 2010.

Bascomb, Neal. *Hunting Eichman*. Houghton Mifflin Harcourt, 2009.

Battin, Margaret Pabst, *Ending Life: Ethics and the Way We Die*. New York: Oxford University Press, 2005.

Bloch, S., and S. Green. *Psychiatric Ethics*, 4th ed. New York: Oxford University Press, 2009.

Bok, Sissela. "Euthanasia." In *Euthanasia and Physician Assisted Suicide*, by G. Dworkin, R. Frey, and S. Bok, chapter 7. Cambridge: Cambridge University Press, 1998.

Burleigh, Michael. *Death and Deliverance: "Euthanasia" in Germany 1900–1945*. Cambridge: Cambridge University Press, 1944.

Carney, D., and S. Horton-Deutsh. "Suicide Over 60: The San Diego Study." *J Am Geriatr Soc.* 42, no. 2 (February 1994): 174–80.

Cassell, Eric J. *Doctoring: The Nature of Primary Care Medicine*. New York: Oxford University Press, 1997.

Cavanaugh, J. T., A. Carson, M. Sharpe, and S. Lawrie. "Psychological Autopsy Studies of Suicide: A Systematic Review." *Psychol Med* 33 (2003): 395–403.

Christakis, N., and E. Lamont. "Extent and Determinations of Error in Doctors Prognosis in Terminally Ill Patients." *BMJ* 320 (February 19, 2000): 469–73.

Churchill, Winston. *Their Finest Hours*. Boston: Houghton, Mifflin, 1999.

Diamond, John. Introduction. In *Because Cowards Get Cancer Too*. New York: Times Books, 1998.

Donne, John. Quote in preface. *For Whom the Bell Tolls*, by Ernest Hemingway. New York: P. F. Collier and Son, 1940.

Dormer, N., K. McCaul, and L. Kristjanson. "Risk of Suicide in Cancer Patients in Western Australia 1981–2002." *Med J Aust* 188, no. 3 (2008): 140–43.

Dworkin, Gerald, R. Frey, and Sissela Bok. *Euthanasia and Physician-Assisted Suicide.* Cambridge: Cambridge University Press, 1998.

Eagle, C. C., et al., "Trends in the Aggressiveness of Cancer Care Near the End of Life." *J Clin Oncol* 22 (2004): 315–21 [PMID: 14722041].

Edwards, B. K., H. L. Howe, L. A. Ries, M. H. Thun, H. M. Rosenberg, R. Yancik, P. A. Wingo, A. Jermal, and E. G. Feigal. "Annual Report to the Nation on the Status of Cancer 1973–1999." *Cancer,* 94, no. 10 (2002): 2766–92.

Emanuel, F. J., Y. Young-Xu, N. G. Levinsky, G. Gazelle, O. Saynina, and A. S. Ash. "Chemotherapy Use Among Medicare Beneficiaries at the End of Life." *Ann Inter Med.* 138 (2003): 639–43 [PMID: 12693886].

Euripides. As quoted from *Bartlett's Famous Quotations*, 15th ed., 77.22. New York: Little, Brown, 1980.

Fazel, S., J. Cartwright, A. Nott-Norman, and K. Hawton. "Suicide in Prisoners: A Systematic Review of Risk Factors." *J Clin Psychiatry* 69 (2008):1721–31.

Furton, E. J., P. Cataldo, and O. Andmoraczewski. *Catholic Health Care Ethics: A Manual for Practitioners*, 2nd ed. Philadelphia, PA: National Catholic Bioethics Center, 2009.

Gajalakshmim V., and R. Peto. "Suicide Rates in Rural Tamil Nadu, South India: Verbal Autopsy of 39,000 Deaths in 1997–98." *Int. J. Epidemiol* 36 (2007): 203–7.

Gallagher, Hugh Gregory. *By Trust Betrayed.* Arlington, VA: Vandamere Press, 1995.

Goodwin, F., and K. Jamison. *Manic-Depressive: Bipolar Disorders and Recurrent Depression*, 2nd ed. New York: Oxford University Press, 2007.

Groopman, Jerome. *The Anatomy of Hope.* New York: Random House, 2005.

Harwood, Michal, et al. "Life Problems and Physical Illness as Risk Factors for Suicide in Older People: A Descriptive Case-Control Study." *Psychol Med.* 36, no. 9 (September 2006): 1265–74.

Holland, Jimmie, and Sheldon Lewis. *The Human Side of Cancer: Living with Hope, Coping with Uncertainty.* New York: HarperCollins, 1999.

Howard, R., P. Inskip, and L. Travis. "Suicide after Childhood Cancer." *J Clin Oncol* 25 (2009):731.

Huxley, Aldous. *Brave New World.* Garden City, NY: Doubleday, 1932.

Jefferson, Thomas. Letter to John Adams, October 28, 1813. In *The Life and Selected Writings of Jefferson*, ed. Adrienne Kock and William Peden, p. 632. New York: Random House, 1944.

Johnson, Tim. "Columbia High Court Approves Mercy Killing." *Boston Globe*, May 22, 1997, 7.

Kass, Leon. *Life, Liberty and the Defense of Dignity.* New York: Encounter Books, 2002.

Kendal, W. "Suicide and Cancer: A Gender-Comparative Study." *Ann Oncol* 18 (2007): 381–87.

King, M., J. Semlyen, S. Seetai, et al. "A Systematic Review of Mental Disorder, Suicide, and Deliberate Self-Harm in Lesbian, Gay and Bisexual People." *BMC Psychiatry* 8 (August 18, 2008): 70.

Kluger, Jeffrey. "How Faith Can Heal." *Time* (February 23, 2009).

Levi, F., C. Lavecchia, F. Lucchini, et al. "Trends in Mortality from Suicide, 1965–99." *Acta Psychiatr Scand.* 108, no. 5 (November 2003): 341–49.

Li, G. "The Interaction Effect of Bereavement and Sex on the Risk of Suicide in the Elderly: An Historic Cohort Study." *Social Science and Medicine* 40 (1995): 825–28.

Llorente, M., M. Burke, C. Gregory, et al. "Prostate Cancer: A Significant Risk Factor for Late-Life Suicide." *Am J. Geriatr Psychiatry* 13, no. 3 (2005):195–201.

Machiavelli, Niccolo. *The Prince.* New York: Oxford University Press, 1998.

Medicare Payment Advisory Commission. "Medicare Payments for Outpatients Drugs under Part B." In *Report to the Congress: Variation and Innovation in Medicare,* chapter 9, June 2005. Accessed at http://www.medpac.gov/publications%5Ccongressional_reports%5CJune03_Ch9.pdf on 17 March 2009.

Miles, S., C. Gomez. *Protocols for Elective Use of Life Sustaining Treatments.* New York: Springer-Verlag, 1988.

Miller, M., H. Mogun, D. Azreal, et al. "Cancer and the Risk of Suicide in Older Americans." *J Clin Oncol* 26, no. 29 (2008): 4720–24.

Merwin, William. Quoted in *Bartlett's Famous Quotations,* 15th ed., p. 907. Little, Brown, 1980.

Morra, Marion, and Eve Potts. *Choices.* New York: Avon Books, 1994.

President's Cancer Panel. *NCI Annual Report, 2004–2005.* Washington, DC: National Cancer Institute.

Nuland, Sherwin, B. *How We Die: Reflections on Life's Final Chapter.* New York: Vintage Books, 1995.

Pendergast, T., and J. M. Luce. "Increasing Incidence of Withholding and Withdrawal of Life Support from the Critically Ill." *Am Journal of Respiratory and Critical Care Medicine* 155, no. 1 (January 1997): 1–2.

Pellegrino, Edmund D. "The John Conley Lecture." Delivered to the Annual Meeting of the American Academy of Otolaryngology / Head and Neck Surgery, San Diego, CA, September 8, 1990.

Philips, M. R., X. Li, and Y. Zhang. "Suicide Rates in China, 1995–99." *Lancet* 359 (2002): 835–40.

Pirl, W., and A. Roth. "Diagnosis and Treatment of Depression in Cancer Patients." *Oncology* 13, no. 9 (1999): 1293–1301.

President's Commission for the Study of Ethical Problems in Medicine and Biomedical and Behavioral Research. "Deciding to Forego Life-Sustaining Treatment." Washington, DC: U.S. Government Printing Office, 1983.

Rasic, D., S. Belik, J. Bolton, et al. "Cancer, Mental Disorders, Suicidal Ideations, and Attempts in a Large Community Sample." *Psycho-Oncology* 17 (2008): 660–67.

Recklitis, C., R. Lockwood, M. Rothwell, et al. "Suicidal Ideation and Attempts in Adult Survivors of Childhood Cancer." *J Clin Oncol* 24, no. 24 (2006): 3852–57.

Resnick, M. "Protecting Adolescents from Harm: Findings from the National Longitudinal Study on Adolescent Health." *JAMA* (September 1997): 823–32.

Russell, Bertrand. *The Autobiography of Bertrand Russell.* New York: Routledge, 2000.

Santayana, George. Quoted in *Bartlett's Famous Quotations,* 15th ed., p. 703. Little, Brown, 1980.

Seneca, Annaeus. Excerpts from Letter 70 in the series of Letters to Lucilius. In *The Stoic Philosophy of Seneca*, ed. and trans. Moses Hadas. New York: W.W. Norton, 1958.

Singh, Kathleen Dowling. *The Grace in Dying*. New York: HarperCollins, 1998.

Smith, Thomas. "Cancer Care: A Microcosm of the Problems Facing All of Health Care."*Annuals of Internal Medicine* 150, no. 8 (2009): 573–76.

Sprung, C. L. "Changing Attitudes and Practices in Forgoing Life Sustaining Treatments." *JAMA* 263 (1990): 2213.

Ubel, Peter. "Cancer Care: A Microcosm of the Problems Facing All of Health Care." *Annals of Internal Medicine* 150, no. 8 (April 22, 2009): 573.

U.S. Census Bureau. *Current Population Report*. Washington, DC: U.S. Census Bureau, 1993.

Waern, M., et al. "Burden of Illness and Suicide in Elderly People: A Case-Control Study." *BMJ* 24, no. 7350 (June 8, 2002): 1355–57.

Walter, Scott. Quote from *The New Dictionary of Thoughts*, ed. Tryon Edwards, rev. and enl. by C. N. Catrevas, Jonathan Edwards, and Ralph Emerson Browns, p. 279. New York: Standard Book Company, 1961.

Wilson, Jennifer Fisher. "Editorial on Cancer Care: A Microcosm of the Problems Facing All of Health Care." *Annals of Int Medicine* 150, no. 8 (2009): 573.

Winawer, Sidney. Quoted on cover of Holland and Lewis, *The Human Side of Cancer*. New York: Harper's, 1999.

World Health Organization. *World Report on Violence and Health*. Geneva, Switzerland: World Health Organization, 1989.

World Health Organization. *World Report on Violence and Health*. Geneva, Switzerland, World Health Organization, 2002.

Index

abandonment, 166–68, 177, 184

abortion, 53–54; desensitization to, 61–62; fetal harm and, 62–63; Hippocratic Oath on, 52–53, 56; as killing, 61–63; physician bias on, 56–58, 67–68; point of viability and, 60–61; psycho-metabolic forces and, 64–65; rarity of necessity of, 63; religious views on, 59–60, 62–63, 66–67; *Roe v. Wade* on, 59, 61–62. *See also* pregnancy

Adams, John, 41, 42, 44, 61, 88

afterlife, 29, 153, 176, 180

age: breast cancer and, 159; culture and, 141–42; death and, 175–76; ignorance and, 151; pregnancy and, 67–68; stigma of, 142–44

"all's clear," 22

alpha oncologist, 25, 94–95, 165, 174, 178

alternative medicine, 113; damage caused by, 145–46; fads in, 145–46; patience with, 144–45; researching, 146; traditional Chinese, 145; translators advocating, 147–48

The Anatomy of Hope (Groopman), 26–27

anesthesiology, 138–40

Annals of Internal Medicine, 32, 161

appendicitis, 42

Archimedes, 49

aristocracy, natural, 8, 11

Armstrong, Lance, 38

arrogance, 18–19, 112–13, 114, 131; avoiding, 102, 119–20, 121

Ars Moriendi (*The Art of Dying*), 180

assisted suicide. *See* suicide

astrology, 52

Aurelius, Marcus, 69

autonomy, patient: in death, 85–86, 97, 155–56; ethics and, 57–59, 68, 69–70, 85–86; informed consent in, 81–82, 118, 155–57, 171–72; stigma and, 142–44

Bascomb, Neal, 75

Battin, Margaret Pabst, 85–86

Because Cowards Get Cancer Too (Diamond), 18

beneficence, patient, 55–57

Binding, Karl, 77

bioethics, 44

birth control. *See* pregnancy

Black, Shirley Temple, 38, 142

bloodletting, 39

Bok, Sissela, 81–82

About the Author

Roy B. Sessions, MD, retired from active practice in 2008 and is currently a professor of Otolaryngology Head and Neck Surgery at the Medical University of South Carolina. He serves as a consultant and attending surgeon at the Ralph H. Johnson Veterans Administration Hospital in Charleston. He has retained his affiliation with Georgetown University School of Medicine as an adjunct professor. During his almost 40-year career he has been responsible for over 140 scientific publications, including three editions of *Cancer of the Head and Neck: A Multidisciplinary Approach* (with Harrison and Hong). The first of these won the Doody International Medical Book of the Year Award among 4,000 other textbooks. He has been associated with the Baylor College of Medicine, Memorial Sloan-Kettering Cancer Center/Cornell Medical College and Beth Israel Cancer Center/Albert Einstein College of Medicine in New York City and served ten years as the chairman of the Department of Otolaryngology—Head and Neck Surgery at Georgetown University School of Medicine. During his academic career, he served as a consultant to the NCI and was a member of the editorial board of their journal, the PDQ. Doctor Sessions has lectured extensively in the United States and internationally, including Germany, China, United Kingdom, Italy, France, Ecuador, Brazil, and Japan.